PAST FOODS

Rediscovering Indigenous and Traditional Crops for Food Security and Nutrition

Kukuwa Abba

Kuumba Books

First published 2021 by Kuumba Books

Image Credits:
Breadfruit and palm trees against Caribbean sky: Fando972 (Pixabay); *African Locust bean flowers*: Ji-Elle (Feedipedia); *Amaranth grain*: Miiya (Pixabay); *Bambara in the field*: Kkibumba (Wikimedia); *Baobab fruit (split/whole)*, *Millets*: T.K. Naliaka (Wikimedia); *Breadfruit*: PublicDomainPictures (Pixabay); *Breadnut fruit*: Dinesh Valke (Flickr); *Breadnut seed*: Bobjgalindo (Wikimedia); *Coconut*: Josch13 (Pixabay); *Eddoe tubers*: RoySmith (Wikimedia); *Taro tubers*: varintorn (Pixabay); *Cowpea plant*: Harry Rose (Wikimedia); *Detar tree with fruit, Detar flowers, Shea fruit*: Marco Schmidt (Wikimedia); *Fonio*: kelson (Wikimedia); *Gungo pea pods*: David E Mead (Wikimedia); *Gungo peas*: C.L. Ramjohn (Wikimedia); *Jackfruit*: balouriarajesh (Pixabay); *Lablab beans*: (Denis Bastianelli) Feedipedia; *Lablab flowers*: কামরুল ইসলাম শাহীন (Wikimedia); *Lablab pods*: Dinesh Valke (Wikimedia); *Finger millet*: Naksh (Pixahive); *Pearl millet*: Sarangib (Maxipixel); *Moringa (ground)*: gensudesleben (Maipixel); *Stinking toe tree*: Forest and Kim Starr (Wikimedia); *Tamarind seeds*: Bhaskaranaidu (Wikimedia); *African sunset*: Ron Porter (Pixabay); *View of the Sahel*: bory67 (Pixabay); Jackfruit (peeled): kieutruongphoto (Pixabay); *Maps of African Sahel and Caribbean Regions*: adapted by Debbie McGowan; *Moringa pods, Tamarind chutney and drink*: licensed images.

All other images copyright © Kukuwa Abba

ISBN number: 978 1 78645 484 3

Edited and typeset by Beaten Track Publishing
Burscough, Lancashire, United Kingdom
Website: www.beatentrackpublishing.com

Acknowledgements

I want to give thanks to HIM Haile Selassie1 for inspiration, guidance and the Blue Print. Thanks to my ancestors for their endurance and their legacy, especially to my mother Normadel Rodgers, who inspired my interest in our food heritage. Thanks to my children: Amina, Isatu, Meshak, Zanya and Eshe and my grandchildren, for love and light. Big thanks to my husband Sazi Fareye, the real Earth Guardian, without whom this book wouldn't have happened. Foofo sanne to my Sahelian son Ali Diallo, Inna really hopes there will be a better future.

More thanks to all my sistren, who have supported the works over the years, with special big-ups to Aya Passley (The Resilient Fern), Sancha Zebi, Margrit Lienert, Danielle Hoogenboom, Dr Imani Tafari-Ama, Nanny Ivey, Kelley Maki and Sydoney Massop. Thanks too to all the farmers across the world, the backbone of the nations, especially those in the West African Sahel and the Caribbean, still cultivating the land, despite the challenges.

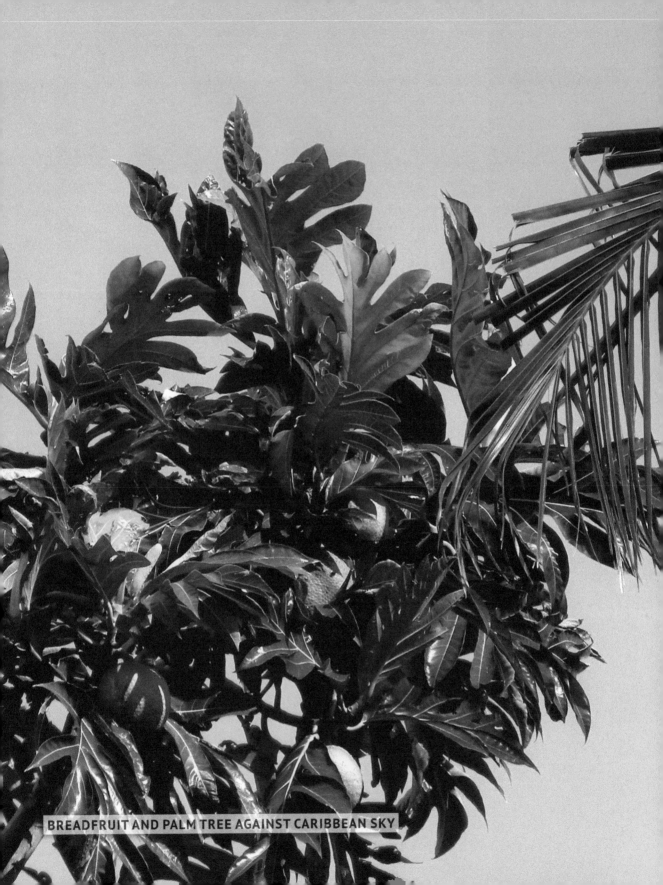

BREADFRUIT AND PALM TREE AGAINST CARIBBEAN SKY

CONTENTS

Even in this nuclear age, in spite of the revolutionary changes in man's life which science has brought about, the problem of further improving and perfecting agricultural methods continues to hold a position of high priority for the human race. A country and a people that become self-sufficient by the development of agriculture can look forward with confidence to the future.

HIM Haile Selassie1 (16.01.1958)

Introduction

Food is the 'staff of life', 'our daily bread', the basis of our energy and nutritional needs. Although central to our very existence, food also plays an important role in social, economic and cultural aspects of our lives. Having enough to eat is still, however, a constant challenge for more than 25% of the world's population. According to the most recent report on the global state of food insecurity (SOFI), at least two billion people are experiencing varying degrees of food insecurity.

The close correlation between a healthy diet and good health means that focused efforts have to be made to ensure that this most basic of human needs is met universally. The current situation, as detailed in the SOFI Report, paints a picture of long-standing and worsening inequalities in access to regular healthy meals. Across the world, food production, distribution and consumption are driven not by people's nutritional needs but more often by greed along the food chain.

The COVID-19 pandemic has again brought the issue of food insecurity and its inevitable consequences to the fore. The dramatic decline in economic activity and subsequent loss of income in addition to disruptions in global supply chains have occurred on an unprecedented scale. The pandemic has amplified the many inequalities and inequities, which have been left unchecked or only feebly and sporadically challenged. Loss of lives and other negative outcomes are therefore unsurprising for those communities, who have consistently featured in national and international misery statistics for decades.

Before COVID-19, the world was grappling with the issue of climate change and the negative effects this was having on already vulnerable regions and their populations. The continued increase in temperatures and changes in weather patterns had already led to scarcity of water, arable lands, pasture lands, forests, semi-forest lands and mangroves.

The roots of many of the social and economic problems, including civil conflicts, particularly in low- and middle-income countries, can be traced to changes in lifestyles impacted by climatic and environmental forces, and their consequences. In East Africa and to a lesser extent parts of Asia, in the past year, there have also been unusually large and persistent swarms of locusts, which have devoured vast swathes of cultivation and added to other existing food insecurity problems.

My interest in food security is rooted in my international health and development experience. The lack of connectivity between the experts promoting the contribution that healthy diets make to overall health improvement and the experts in agriculture and food security was a constant source of frustration. Despite policies and initiatives to improve 'joined-up approaches', there continue to be significant gaps between these important areas of the Sustainable Development Goals (SDGs). The problems of access and affordability are the main issues, and these have to be addressed in the context of the food systems that produce and market food and the wider social, economic and cultural environment.

Over the past decade, I have witnessed, first-hand, developments in some of the vulnerable countries in the Sahel region of West Africa, where food insecurity, initially caused by climate and environmental changes, has been worsened by human activities. Widespread violence by armed groups has only compounded the situation, and this has resulted in a vicious cycle of civil conflicts, population displacement and greater food insecurity.

Contrasting the situation in those countries and comparing it to my native Jamaica and other Caribbean islands, I realised that despite the obvious differences between these two regions, they face many similar challenges. In their different ways, they exemplify ecological and other vulnerabilities that affect various parts of the world.

The Sahel is perhaps the worst example of rapid desertification anywhere on Earth, and what happens there should be a salutary lesson for other arid and semi-arid regions. The Caribbean region is at the mercy of an annual hurricane season that lasts from June to November. Depending on the force of the particular storm, there can be serious natural and infrastructural destruction, all of which has economic, social and health implications.

Although the Caribbean might have higher average income levels than many countries in West Africa, they mask significant inequalities within the population. Tourism and high rates of remittances from Caribbean migrants have perhaps masked fundamental weaknesses in these island economies, but sudden economic shocks reveal their frailties. The current fallout from COVID-19 is set to exacerbate an already fragile situation and increase food insecurity, especially for low-income groups.

We know that just having more food is not the same as having a healthy diet, and any efforts to address the challenges of accessing more nutritious food will also have to include the provision of information to improve knowledge about nutrition in the population at large. The hope is that if more people know about the benefits of different foods, the more likely they will be to prioritise the cultivation, storage, processing and preparation of foods most suited to meeting their nutritional needs.

According to botanists, there are more than 400,000 plant species on Earth, with about half of these being potentially edible for humans. A review of the food crops currently being used in the world concluded that about 200 species are known to be consumed, but fewer than 20 species now provide 90% of our foods. More alarming is the fact that three (3) crops – maize, rice and wheat – provide more than half of the calories and proteins derived from plants.

Clearly, we are not making use of the range of plants available to us for food. If there is such large-scale food insecurity in the world, it would make sense to halt or at least reduce the reliance on the crops we currently depend on. We need to widen our scope and include other crops that can contribute to increasing the number of people who can afford to consume a healthy diet. For those living in the Sahel and other parts of Sub-Saharan Africa and on vulnerable islands in the Caribbean, more efforts need to be made to explore what is available where they are, as well as what is possible to grow locally without expensive, imported inputs.

Some of these crops have been described as 'orphan' or 'lost' crops and the main mission of *Past Foods* is to promote the benefits of rediscovering these crops for improving food security and making diets healthier. We know from long experience, however, that even when there is information and provision, people still choose what they eat by preference and habit. It is not easy to change behaviours, attitudes and practice with information alone; other strategies are needed to get individuals and groups to prioritise their food choices based primarily on nutritional needs.

West Africa and the Caribbean share a long history over many centuries, mostly defined by the transatlantic trade in enslaved Africans. Even today, there are many lasting social, economic and cultural legacies in both Africa and the New World, from that experience. One of the most interesting and important is the botanical legacy: the introduction of species from Africa to the Americas and vice versa.

Most of the crops included in *Past Foods* fall into this category, and the history and movements of these crops reflect in many ways our own journeys, the most important of which is to recognise the value of crops, which have survived so much, and to consume them in a sustainable way. All the crops in *Past Foods* have been around for thousands of years and still have the characteristics to be regarded as 'superfoods', despite their 'low social and economic status' in some cases.

Environmental issues are major considerations when addressing agricultural development, and climate-smart approaches to improving food security are important, as is water and the key role it plays in all aspects of food from cultivation to preparation. Scarcity of water, therefore, has major implications for increasing agricultural production and improving diets and overall health.

Past Foods aims to provide some background information on current food systems in which large-scale mono-crop production models are seen as the answer to food security issues. This is contrasted with more sustainable approaches that can deliver results while preserving biodiversity and improving rural development.

Information on the ways in which a healthy diet can improve health, well-being and overall development is briefly summarised. The rationale for the choice of the particular crops is briefly outlined before the individual crops are featured. For those who want to try some of the foods in the book, there are a few suggested recipes that will hopefully whet the appetite and encourage readers to create their own.

Additional material is provided in the Appendices for those who want to know more about some of the issues touched on in the book, including a brief section on aspects of nutrition that will help to underpin the information provided throughout the book.

In the spirit of the West African concept of 'Sankofa', we are rediscovering foods from the past, which will help us face the present and future reality of food insecurity.

'Se wo were fi na wosankofa a yenki' (Twi)

'It is not wrong to go back for what you've forgotten'

PAST FOODS

Background

In 2015, at the United Nations General Assembly, member states adopted 17 Sustainable Development Goals (SDGs), which were to provide a blueprint for peace, progress and prosperity for the people and the planet. For many people working in international development, despite some scepticism, it seemed that there might finally be a coherent framework, which governments could adapt to reflect local needs and circumstances. These goals were to be achieved by 2030, an ambitious aim, given the starting point for some countries. For others working in development, neither the goals nor the timeline was ambitious enough.

Zero Hunger is the headline goal for SDG 2, by ensuring access to safe, nutritious and sufficient food for all people, all year round. It also aims to eradicate all forms of malnutrition, which include stunting, wasting, overweight and obesity. The achievement of SDG 2 necessitates increased agricultural production, while ensuring that these increases are environmentally sustainable.

It is now five years on, and it is clear from the latest State of Food Security and Nutrition in the World (SOFI) Report that ending hunger, increasing food security and improving nutrition are not on course to be achieved and future trends do not look promising. Current estimates suggest that in 2019, more than two billion people, or 25% of the world's population, either experienced hunger or did not have regular access to sufficient food.

The majority of those experiencing food insecurity live in Asia, but Sub-Saharan Africa has the highest percentage by population and the fastest growing rates. As expected, food insecurity is strongly related to poverty, and the highest rates are in low-income countries, and although middle- and higher-income countries have fewer numbers, they too have vulnerable, food-insecure communities. Many factors can contribute to food insecurity: conflicts; extreme weather events; climate change; infrastructural inadequacies; and as seen recently, unforeseen events such as the COVID-19 global pandemic and the locust swarms which have been plaguing parts of East Africa in the past year.

It is the unforeseen, novel COVID-19, which has had the most widespread and dramatic impacts on lives and livelihoods globally. As this is an evolving situation, it is still to be seen just how far-reaching the damage will be, but the SOFI Report estimates that 80–120 million more people could become food insecure in the coming months as a result of the health and socioeconomic impacts of COVID-19.

The theme of the 2020 SOFI Report is: Transforming Food Systems for Affordable Healthy Diets. For the purposes of this book, a healthy diet is defined in concurrence with WHO as:

> A diet which contains a balanced, diverse and appropriate selection of foods eaten over a period of time.

Analysis of the true cost of eradicating malnutrition showed that the cost of a healthy diet exceeds the $1.90, which is seen as a minimum requirement per person, per day. In fact, more than 50% of people living in Sub-Saharan Africa and South Asia cannot afford what is defined as a healthy diet, and these are the same places where food insecurity rates are highest.

Even in more developed economies, there are many people who cannot afford the cost of a healthy diet, and just as it is in developing countries, if people cannot afford healthy diets, they are likely to become malnourished, whether by lack of food or consuming too much of the wrong type of food, resulting in either wasting or overweight and obesity.

These manifestations of malnutrition caused by unhealthy diets need to be addressed, but how? Transforming current food systems is complex, political and subject to unexpected shocks and reversals. In recent decades, transnational agribusiness corporations have been favoured at the expense of small farmers, who actually produce 70% of the food consumed in places like Africa. There is no doubt that technological advances in agriculture have brought significant benefits to billions of people, but many of these methods have proven to be detrimental to human and animal health and have cost the Earth in many ways.

Despite the growing evidence of these negative impacts and lingering misgivings, international governmental organisations, donor organisations and private sector interests continue to fund and support policies and investments that are detrimental to small farmers, especially those in some of the most food-insecure parts of the world. These powerful players are convinced that their approaches are the best way to eradicate hunger, increase food security and improve nutrition.

In the past decade, two initiatives focusing on Africa have again demonstrated that top-down, large-scale projects are still being imposed on the continent as part of strings-attached aid programmes, which run counter to the needs of the farmers and people there. The Alliance for a Green Revolution in Africa (AGRA), funded by the Gates Foundation, the Rockefeller Foundation and with additional funds from various governmental aid agencies, was established in 2006 to bring about an agricultural revolution in Africa. The Alliance's main aim was to increase incomes and improve food security for 30 million small-holder farm households by 2021.

Taking a technological approach, with widespread use of high-yield commercial seeds, chemical fertilisers and pesticides, AGRA aimed to double agricultural productivity and household incomes and reduce by 50% the rates of food insecurity in the 13 countries in which they were to operate. As AGRA nears the deadline for the achievement of its goals, it has not presented any reports which provide data on progress towards or achievement of the stated goals.

Independent evaluations using other data sources have presented a scenario where the number of undernourished people has increased in the 13 countries in which AGRA operates by an average of 30%. There is little evidence of the doubling of yield or incomes for the seven million farmers directly targeted and a further 21 million indirectly targeted in this initiative.

Even when productivity aims were exceeded as in maize production in Zambia, it did not lead to a reduction in poverty or food insecurity, in fact quite the opposite. It seems that AGRA's tag line 'from a solitary struggle to survive to a business that thrives' has remained a distant dream for millions of African farmers.

Another related initiative, the New Alliance for Food Security and Nutrition in Africa (NAFSN) was launched under the auspices of the G8 in 2012. Its aim was to achieve sustained and inclusive agricultural growth and raise 50 million people out of poverty by 2022.

This was to be attained by creating the conditions that would allow the participating countries to improve agricultural productivity and develop their agri-food sector by attracting more private investment in agriculture. Despite widespread criticism and protests from a wide array of experts, civil society groups, farmers' groups and concerned citizens, substantial funds and other inducements were provided to national and multinational agribusiness corporations to support the aims of the initiative.

One of the criticisms levelled at NAFSN was that the reach and interests of companies like Monsanto, Syngenta, Yara, Cargill, Unilever, Diageo and General Mills, among others, were being supported by government funds under the banner of aid to Africa. Under this model, the proposed aid beneficiaries would in the first instance be these private corporations, who would now have a foothold in Africa, in a very unequal partnership.

The glossy public relations material gives the impression that there was not only widespread support from small farmers for NAFSN, but that they were also meaningfully involved in its development. However, if one considers the short-, medium- and long-term implications for these farmers, their agreement to and support of the terms and conditions of the proposals would have been akin to turkeys voting for Thanksgiving.

Ten countries in Africa were chosen for NAFSN intervention, and corporations were given finance, tax incentives, land tenure and rights in order to produce mono crops on an industrial scale. Legislation had to be passed in participating countries to facilitate takeover of large tracts of land by these private corporations and to ensure that the local climate was conducive to business.

Strict laws relating to the ownership and trade of non-certified seeds meant that traditional seed sharing and trading, which had been carried out for millennia, could now be penalised with fines and imprisonment. In Tanzania, the fines were at least $210,000, 12 years' imprisonment or both! Apart from patented seeds, chemical fertilisers and other inputs were tied to multinational corporations, and many farmers found themselves in a cycle of debt, poverty and food insecurity, instead of the wonderful promises of success made to them.

NAFSN received technical and implementation support from AGRA, so there was a lot of synergy in the work they did in the countries in which they operated, and they share many of the same failings. France withdrew from NAFSN early in 2018, citing a review of the programme in Burkina Faso, where it observed the real risks of land grabbing to the detriment of small farmers and pointed to the fact that only an agro-ecological approach could succeed in addressing the development needs of the Sahel region and its people.

Unflattering evaluations from Canadian and other funding agencies have all pointed to the same shortcomings and failures of NAFSN. The Independent Commission for Aid Impact (ICAI) in a review of NAFSN in 2015, stated that the initiative 'had performed relatively poorly against their criteria for effectiveness and value for money'.

Given the negative outcomes of some aspects of the initiative, it has been described as 'Agricultural Colonialism' by Members of the European Union Parliament (MEPs). Monsanto, in an ironic twist, accused the EU of 'neo-colonialism' for not allowing African countries to reap the benefits of genetically modified organism (GMO) technology, despite 'scientific consensus' on its safety. In truth, there is no such consensus, with very strong arguments on both sides of the debate.

Another non-government organisation (NGO) described NAFSN/AGRA as a Trojan Horse for the corporate takeover of African agriculture. It argued that if the same level of incentives and funding were to be used to support small farmers, there would be far better outcomes across most indices, such as yield, income, rural development and empowerment of marginalised groups including women. Another huge downside of these types of initiatives is that they destroy biodiversity, with their emphasis on mono crops, such as corn, soya and rice. The built-in dependence on patented seeds is unacceptable, especially the risk of loss of remaining African species.

It is no surprise that the private companies involved should come up with solutions to Africa's food security problems that have synergy with their own corporate aims. The agricultural models they promote have already come under scrutiny in Europe, in particular the widespread use of GMO seeds and plants. They may be limited in North America by geography and climate, but in recent decades, there have been expansions into Central and South America and in Southeast Asia by many of these same players.

A prime example of this is the Cargill company, whose tag line is 'Helping the world thrive', and they are certainly thriving as one of the largest privately owned conglomerates in the USA. It is estimated that this family has the most billionaires within a family, but as Cargill has no shareholders, the company is not obliged to disclose those figures.

One of their executives once stated that the mission of the company was 'the commercialisation of photosynthesis'. Their public relations are more measured these days, as they present themselves as the solution to the world's food problems. However, a closer look at this food-chain commodity giant shows why efforts to transform food systems are fraught with fundamental difficulties.

Cargill produces grains, oilseeds, soya and cocoa beans and other crops on a huge scale and is involved with every aspect of global food production, but you are unlikely to see their name on a label in your supermarket. Their turnover last year was over $100 billion, with more than 155,000 employees across 70 countries. The sheer scope and reach of their operations are quite startling when you consider that they are fundamentally a private agricultural company.

Over the years, there have been reports of the true cost of their business to the planet and some of its people. Unfortunately, this global giant is known for its reluctance to be in the spotlight; it is therefore not easy to keep track of all of the company's activities.

In Africa, they have been involved in large-scale mono crop production in South Africa, Kenya and Zambia and are heavily involved in the cocoa agribusiness in Ghana, Ivory Coast and Cameroon. Despite their headline phrase, there have been claims and counterclaims as to the extent to which companies, like Cargill are contributing to improvements in nutrition, or reduction in food insecurity in Africa or even helping local communities to thrive.

One of the evaluations of AGRA in East and South East Africa concluded that despite increased maize production in some instances, the high cost of inputs had a negative impact on the household income of small farmers. Worse, however, was that the higher-yield maize had begun to displace traditional crops such as millets and sorghum, which have proven over centuries to be resilient in extreme conditions and have always contributed to food security in that part of the world.

This is and has been a recurring theme across Sub-Saharan African countries, particularly where external entities and agencies have researched the food security problem and decided that the introduction of genetically manipulated crops will be the answer to the food security problems there. Many traditional crops have been marginalised or worse, eradicated due to the introduction of 'better' ones from somewhere else. Loss of seed heritage has had a more significant negative impact than most people realise, and with the loss of seeds, plants and trees, the knowledge associated with them is also lost.

These expensive, multinational, corporate experiments have highlighted the limitations of input-intensive agro-systems and limitations in the ability of these systems to mitigate environmental degradation and adapt to climate change. Large-scale mono crop models of agriculture might have their place in food production, but they have substantial social, economic and environmental costs. Low-cost, low-input approaches, within the context of agro-ecology, can deliver improved yields and sustainable food systems that reduce environmental impacts while offering healthy and nutritious foods.

A report from the EU in 2019 summarised it thus:

> Farmers have again and again proved that they can grow healthy plants and achieve good results, by agro-ecological means, such as intercropping, crop rotation, use of beneficial species and natural soil fertility. Companies that sell pesticides and chemical fertilisers aren't happy if sustainable agricultural practices win ground.

In light of the statement above, it is logical to assume that there would be more resources committed to agro-ecological initiatives across Sub-Saharan Africa, yet the 'Cargill' model of addressing food insecurity and nutrition is growing in influence and scope. By virtue of the inadequacy of investment in agro-ecological programmes in regions like the Sahel, some NGOs have continued with their efforts to improve the conditions there and address the many challenges in achieving food security in sustainable ways.

Nutrition and Health

Under-nutrition is a serious issue, and its effects are worse on the poor, the aged, women and children. Sometimes referred to as 'hidden hunger', it contributes to almost 50% of all deaths in under-fives and to the increased frequency, severity and duration of illnesses such as diarrhoea, respiratory infections and malaria. Poor water and sanitation and other environmental factors contribute to under-nutrition by facilitating further infections and intestinal parasites, which in turn reduce the availability of nutrients from the diet.

The main consequences of chronic under-nutrition, particularly in the vulnerable groups referred to above, are protein energy malnutrition (PEM), which is a macro-nutrient deficiency, and micronutrient malnutrition (MM). Marasmus and Kwashiorkor are the most severe forms of PEM and are indicative of inadequate protein, carbohydrates and fats in the diet. The main micronutrients which are deficient in MM are vitamins A, C and E, and the minerals iron and iodine, with others such as zinc, calcium and B vitamins being important for pregnant and lactating women and infants.

The other aspect of malnutrition is overweight and obesity, which have been rising across all regions of the world, with the greatest rates of increase in middle-income countries and even among the middle classes of low-income countries. Increases in the importation of food have led to changes in food choices, with a shift away from traditional root crops, fruits and vegetables to processed foods that are energy-dense and high in fats, sugars and salt.

The marketing strategies for many imported products convey messages of being more nutritious and better quality than local foodstuff, and as such are seen as being something that people should aspire to consume. There is little doubt that changes in other areas of modern, urban lifestyles have led to reduced physical activity, which also contributes to overweight and obesity.

Overweight and obesity can lead to significant increase in the prevalence and incidence of diseases such as high blood pressure (hypertension), diabetes, heart disease, various cancers, respiratory and musculoskeletal conditions. It is estimated that increases in these non-communicable diseases (NCDs) will add to the burden of infectious diseases that exist in many developing countries and will put further pressure on already inadequate healthcare services.

All countries in the Caribbean region have higher than average rates of overweight and obesity and, unsurprisingly, higher than average rates of NCDs. In the Sahel and some other parts of West Africa, there are variations in the rates of NCDs, with higher rates in urban areas. The challenge in many West African and other medium- and low-income countries is how to tackle ongoing high levels of infectious, communicable diseases and undernourishment as well as increasing rates of overweight among some sections of their population.

Reducing rates of overweight and obesity has proved difficult to achieve, even in well-resourced countries. Unlike anti-smoking campaigns, where people are asked to give up something that has no other purpose, changing eating behaviours is fraught with difficulties. People have to eat; avoiding food is not an option. In most approaches to weight reduction, the onus is on the individual: it is their responsibility to exercise willpower and control over what they eat. However, professionals working in this field can attest to the fact that making the necessary changes to reduce obesity is not easy, and when they are made, they can be even more difficult to sustain.

Governments can help to make the overall social environment less 'obesogenic', by limiting the availability of the wrong types of food or making it easier to afford healthier options. They can enact legislation and propose policies that can increase the production and availability of whole grains, fruits and vegetables or increase taxes on unhealthy processed foods, particularly those that are imported.

Food security is the first step in protecting the health and development of the people, having access to the quantity, quality and variety of foodstuff that will provide the range of micro- and macronutrients that are needed for daily human function. In tandem with increased access to affordable healthy foods, information and advice around nutrition have to be more widely available at a systematic level, for everyone.

Ways have to be found to communicate what consuming a healthy diet looks like, and what the most likely sources of those nutrients are, especially in the context of what grows locally. Technology can contribute to this process in ways that were not feasible a decade ago. Regardless of educational status, new media has the potential to entice, inform, influence and motivate large groups and populations on a given issue.

The golden rule of health literacy and other initiatives for transformation is to begin with what is already known by those most involved: local knowledge is crucial. If this were done consistently, there would be fewer failures in development programmes. Nutrition and its role in health has to be central to how crops are prioritised, cultivated, processed and stored. In the regions of my focus, the West African Sahel and the Caribbean, there is enormous latent potential in revisiting traditional and indigenous knowledge and practice related to various crops, which for one reason or another are not being best utilised, given their nutritional profile.

Summary of the Situation in the Caribbean Region

Almost all the countries in the Caribbean share to a greater or lesser degree the same vulnerabilities to their food supply chains. These are affected by weather events or climate variations, changes in global prices for key commodities that are imported and falls in foreign exchange rates. These factors force governments to make stark choices of what to buy with scarce foreign exchange: food, pharmaceuticals, petroleum supplies?

The dramatic fall in agricultural production in most Caribbean countries has brought huge import bills in its wake. Half of the countries import more than 80% of what they consume, and this equates to an estimated $5 billion annual food import bill for the region. Put that in the context of an over-reliance on the tourism industry and overseas remittances, and the fragilities become readily exposed. The current global pandemic and its attendant threat to lives and livelihoods merely magnifies a chronic, economic ailment that had not been remedied.

Even where there is significant agricultural production, it still tends to follow historical cultivation of sugar cane, bananas and similar crops for export. These islands have limited arable land, in terms of acreage, so policies that continue to encourage the cultivation of crops which neither contribute to national food security and nutrition nor significant foreign exchange earnings have to be revised towards those that offer a level of social protection to local populations in the first instance. Innovative approaches need to be taken in the development of new opportunities in agriculture that can improve food security and nutrition.

The Caribbean is home to a dazzling array of flora, and what is needed is more research and application of results based on local edible species, with a view to developing more widely the production of what are termed 'functional foods'. These have the potential for meeting the nutritional needs of the people in the Caribbean and for exports beyond the region to earn valuable foreign exchange, in a sustainable way.

Summary of the Situation in the West African Sahel

West Africa on the whole has traditionally been more food secure than other parts of the continent. The geography of the region with rainforests, plateaus, savannah and coastal lands and many large rivers, has provided a wide variety of food crops for the people over thousands of years. Even throughout the centuries of devastation caused by the transatlantic trade in enslaved Africans, agricultural traditions were somehow maintained.

Dramatic and rapid changes in the climate and environmental devastation that have occurred in the Sahel region of West Africa have precipitated a chain of events that threaten the region and its people. The desertification of vast swathes of land and the traumatic effects this is having on the land, the animals, the people and their way of life is eye-opening.

The scarcity of water, loss of arable lands for agriculture and animal rearing have led to conflicts, which have escalated, and there are now a variety of insurgencies in the region that have further exacerbated the problems there. Communal clashes between farmers and herdsmen and the many millions now displaced internally by violent conflicts are manifestations of the effects of decades of deteriorating environmental, social and political conditions that had not been adequately addressed.

Countries like Mali, Burkina Faso, Niger and Chad are facing multiple challenges from disrupted farming systems in many areas, internally displaced people and a worsening economic situation compounded by COVID-19 and reductions in remittances from overseas. These factors have led to growing food insecurity, increased malnutrition and high rates of disease and ill health. Given these conditions, zero hunger is not likely, nor is access to healthy diets. Environmental degradation has led to further loss of biodiversity, which can only add to the huge and varied challenges that beset this region.

African Rice – A Cautionary Tale

One of the cautionary tales of abandoned or 'orphan' crops is about African rice, known by its botanical name, Oryza glaberrima, which is related to Asian rice, Oryza sativa. Over thousands of years, O glaberrima developed its own unique features and variations within the African landscape and conditions: there was rice which grew most of the time in water and was planted around inland river deltas, such as the Niger Delta in Mali, rice which grew on drier, upland areas, and rain-fed varieties, all selected over time to suit the local environments and needs.

Like most things in life, African rice had its proponents and its detractors, and when Asian rice was introduced into Africa, the local rice was soon relegated to special occasions and rituals. Admittedly, there were some difficulties associated with its harvesting and milling, and gradually, the easily polished foreign rice displaced African rice, especially the distinctive red rice.

This rice is now only seen in a few parts of the vast areas where many varieties once flourished. The high-yield hybrid rice adopted by farmers began to need more fertilisers and other inputs to produce the same yields as before. Soon, the people could buy cheap imported rice direct from Asia, so the farmers stopped planting rice altogether, except for a few, of course, who were stubborn.

West African rice production was well advanced even before the arrival of Europeans, and the enslaved Africans took their rice grains with them to the New World, whenever possible. The Surinamese Maroons have a legend about the African woman who brought rice to the New World, hidden in her plaits. When the colonial settlers in southeastern states of the USA decided to cultivate rice on a large scale, they turned to the enslaved Africans from Senegambia and Guinea coast, who were skilled rice growers.

In the Caribbean, there are places where rice was cultivated, but most countries import their rice, with the exception of Guyana and Surinam, both of which are located on the South American mainland but associate and identify with the Caribbean rather than Latin America. Rice is one of Guyana's main export crops and is also grown in Surinam, with most commercial production of Asian rice being carried out by people whose ancestors originated or migrated from India and Indonesia.

The Maroons in Suriname are said to still have examples of O glaberrima, which have been traded and exchanged among the various Maroon communities in Guyana and Suriname for centuries. They use the red rice for rituals in much the same way as it was used in West Africa. So now, on both sides of the Atlantic, African rice is being lost, and we are now learning that some of the very features that made it less popular are the ones which make it more nutritious than the other variety. Instead of exploring how to improve the varieties of African rice, increase yields and develop more efficient processing methods, the perceived wisdom from the experts was to introduce more and better varieties of Asian rice.

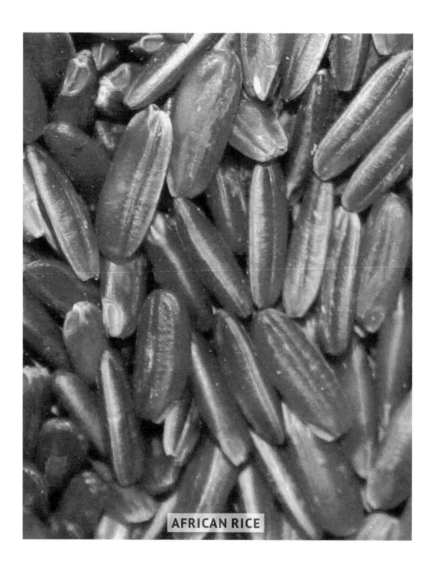

AFRICAN RICE

THE PAST FOODS

Finding ways to alleviate hunger and poverty doesn't always depend on new crop varieties that are based in a laboratory. Instead re-igniting an interest in and a taste for indigenous and traditional foods can help nutrition, increase incomes, restore agricultural biodiversity and preserve local cultures.

Nourish the Planet Team

Experts who work in the area of food and nutrition security agree that reliance on the Big Five – rice, corn, soya, wheat and potatoes – is unsustainable and that the large-scale production of these crops is actually contributing to environmental degradation and climate change. These factors in turn exacerbate food and nutrition insecurity for hundreds of millions of people across the world.

This indicates the need for policy makers, business leaders and social activists to support efforts to advance research that can promote the consumption of a wider variety of foodstuff to improve food and nutrition security. Many of the indigenous food crops that have been classified as 'orphan crops' have nutritional benefits and often do not require the expensive inputs which are required for the Big Five and other more favoured plants. The crops which I have selected for *Past Foods* should be seen primarily as a few examples of the many food crops that exist and whose benefits should be better promoted.

The main geographical focus of this book is the Sahel and the Caribbean Region. However, many of the food crops in *Past Foods* are grown in other parts of the world with similar climatic and geographical conditions, such as South and Central America, parts of Asia and the Pacific region.

With most policy emphasis being on mono crops for export and domestic use, there has been little interest in the research and development of most indigenous foods. Many of these under-utilised crops might not be traded internationally, but they are well adapted to their local environments and can play a greater role in improving food security.

The tree crops provide a source of additional income, often for women, which can contribute to improved nutrition and socioeconomic conditions. These trees are also good as food sources for a variety of animals, some of which are themselves consumed as food. The trees provide shade for humans and animals, reduce erosion and their leaves help to improve soil condition.

The trees and other plants in *Past Foods* can be part of intercropped systems that maintain biodiversity and naturally reduce some of the pests and diseases that large scale farming methods perpetuate.

The nutritional profile of a particular food crop is an important criterion for inclusion in this book. As mentioned in the 'Nutrition' section, human beings need to have a range of both micro- and macronutrients to meet their physical and other requirements. The more nutrients a particular foodstuff has, the more useful it can be in terms of food security. Thus there are fruits which have seeds that can produce flour and cooking oil and trees that have edible, nutritious leaves, fruits and seeds.

Fruits, nuts and edible seeds are of special importance as they can be consumed out of hand or preserved in some way for later use. For many people who are food insecure, especially those who have become food insecure due to natural disaster or civil conflict, having something nutritious to eat that does not require preparation or cooking is vital to their survival.

Data suggest that in many of the countries facing food insecurity, a lot of food is lost post-harvest due to poor handling, transportation issues and inadequate storage. It is therefore important to identify and promote crops that have characteristics and properties which give them a long shelf life or have the ability to retain their overall quality and nutritive value for a prolonged period.

Rediscovering traditional indigenous food crops is only the first stage in the journey because it is important that these foods are acceptable and available to those people who need them. Unfortunately, research has shown that even where a particular food is available and nutritious, it does not necessarily follow that it is going to be accepted, even by those who need it. Taste, preference and habit are more powerful determinants of consumption patterns.

Most of our preferences are shaped by familiarity, what we have become used to. New things do not become accepted overnight, it usually takes time even when the 'new' things have been around far longer than newer, more widely available foodstuffs.

Everything, including cultural practices, is subject to change and evolution, so the first steps have to be taken, and hopefully, the momentum of the necessity for change in local and global patterns of agricultural production, food distribution and consumption patterns will increase.

In the course of gathering the information in the book, it struck me just how many of these crops would be classified in the healthy eating marketing jargon as 'superfoods'. Comparing them with internationally available products that are promoted as such, they are not only comparable but, in some cases, surpass the nutritive benefits of currently available superfoods.

Some of these crops could become the next heavily marketed 'big thing', but hopefully, they won't follow the downsides of the success that quinoa has enjoyed as a super-grain. On the face of it, the popularity of the grain should be a good thing for the people who produce it, but unfortunately, increased international demand has contributed to increased prices for quinoa, putting it out of reach of many for whom it has long been a traditional staple crop.

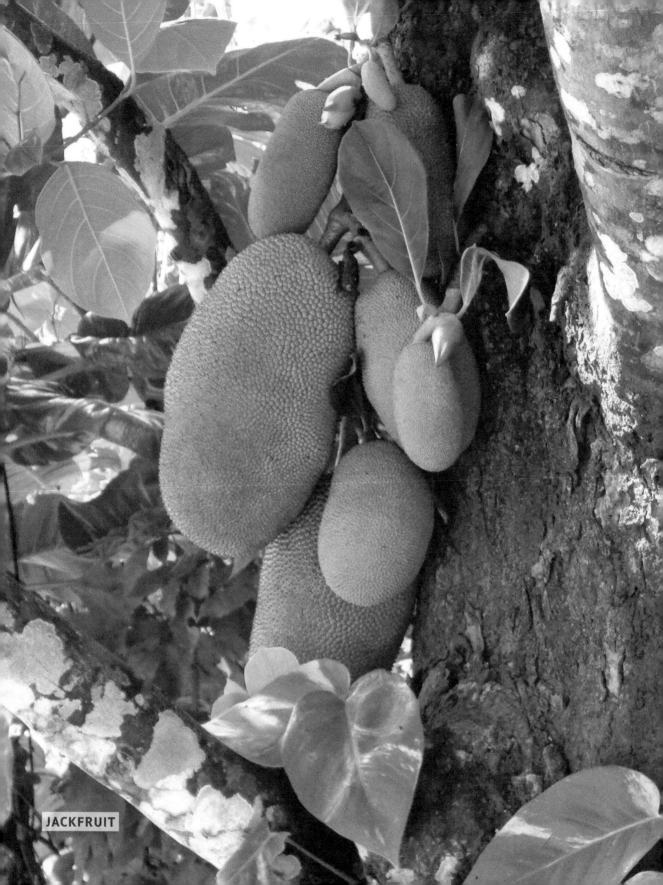
JACKFRUIT

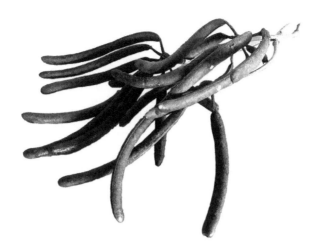

African Locust Bean

Local Names: *Dawadawa; Nere; Monkey Cutlass Tree; Netto; Arbre a Farine; Soumbala; Mkunde; Rouaga; Narghi; Dosso; Dours*

Botanical Information: *Parkia biglobosa (Fabaceae)*

The African locust bean tree can reach heights of 20 metres or more and has a large, spreading crown and branches. The bark of the tree is thick and fissured and when cut produces a deep-yellow gum. The dark-green leaves of the African locust bean are fern-like and consist of pairs of leaflets that make up each part of the compound leaves, which can measure up to 30 cms long.

The tree is attractive, especially when in bloom, with bright-red, round flowers hanging on long stalks like shop-bought decorations. Trees start flowering within 5–7 years and can live for up to 100 years. The African locust bean's flowers bear clusters of reddish-brown pods, and these can be up to 40 cms in length and around 2 cms wide, with between 20 and 40 seeds that are covered by a golden-coloured, powdery substance. The flowers are pollinated by a wide variety of insects and bats; the fruits are eaten by baboons and monkeys, the seeds by birds, who in turn also disperse them.

African locust bean grows in a wide swathe across the savannah of Africa, in more than 20 Sub-Saharan African countries. The tree can thrive in a variety of ecological zones from tropical forests to arid areas with low rainfall and can also grow at fairly high altitudes in a variety of soils. Hundreds of thousands of tonnes of African locust bean seeds are collected, processed and traded across West Africa, especially the fermented seed balls, known widely by their Hausa name *dawadawa*.

Food Products

The fresh fruit powder that surrounds the seeds is rich in protein, vitamins and minerals. It is eaten raw, made into drinks or added as a sweetener to other dishes. In many rural parts of Africa where the tree grows, the fruit powder is mixed with grain and milk or water and given to babies and young children. It is also made into a popular, refreshing drink and adds body and flavour to any smoothie or porridge. The powder is pressed into balls or cakes for storage, which can be extremely useful in times of need. African locust bean fruit powder has the potential to become a 'superfood' by itself or as part of functional food products.

The seeds are the most widely used part of the African locust bean and are fermented, dried and made into greasy, black balls, which are grated and added to stews, soups and rice

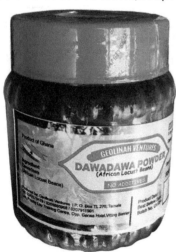

DAWADAWA POWDER

dishes. There are records of this condiment dating as far back as the 14th century. It is rich in protein and other nutrients and is often described as smelling like cheese and having an acquired taste. These balls can be kept in the heat for prolonged periods without refrigeration. Roasted African locust bean seeds can be ground and used as a coffee substitute, known as Sudan coffee or *café negre*.

Although African locust bean and its products are mainly traded across West Africa, with the increase in the number of people of West African heritage living in Europe and North America, the dried, fermented seeds are being traded further from their source and in growing quantities. African locust bean continues to be of social, economic and cultural importance, wherever it grows, and its potential to contribute to food and nutrition security could see increasing demand for its various products.

Medicinal Properties

With the high levels of nutrients in the fruit powder, African locust bean has an important role to play in reducing health conditions and diseases related to nutritional deficiencies, such as vitamin A deficiency (VAD). It can also help to improve immunity and overall health with its vitamins, minerals and fibre.

Most parts of the tree are used for medicinal purposes, wherever it grows. The twigs are chewed and used to clean teeth and to make a mouthwash. The bark is taken internally for fevers including malaria, chest problems such as bronchitis, gastric conditions including vomiting and diarrhoea as well as externally

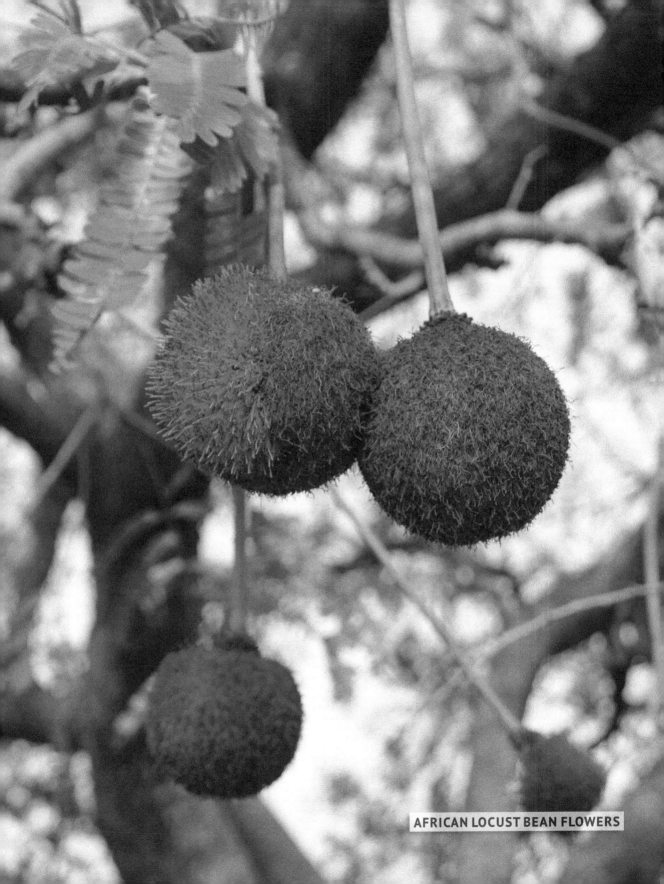

AFRICAN LOCUST BEAN FLOWERS

for skin infections. The leaves are used to treat burns, haemorrhoids and skin conditions.

Other Uses

The African locust bean tree acts as a windbreak and provides much-needed shade for humans and livestock. The urine and dung of the animals plus the leaf fall contribute to ongoing soil improvement, and people collect the leaves to use as a fertiliser generally, as they are rich in nitrogen and minerals.

History/Lore

The botanical name for this tree, *Parkia biglobosa*, is in honour of Mungo Park, a Scottish surgeon and naturalist, who set out to explore the course of the Niger River in West Africa in the 1790s. Park was the first European to record the African locust bean tree, and the botanical name was in recognition of this.

The African locust bean is found on many Caribbean islands, where the tree has become naturalised since being brought there during the course of the Atlantic slave trade. Effective use of the tree and its fruits does not seem to be prevalent, and it is regarded mainly as an ornamental and shade tree. The potential for better use of African locust bean in the region exists and should be explored more rigorously, especially in light of increasing drought in the Caribbean.

In some parts of the African savannah, where the tree grows, it is often one of only three or four trees that can thrive in those environments, baobab, shea and desert date being the others. So important are these trees that in several West African countries, there are laws against cutting them down. African locust bean tree is so reliable in its annual fruiting, even where there has been drought, that in Muslim tradition in the Sahel, it is described as a gift from heaven.

Nutrition Information

Part of Plant	Protein	Carbohydrates	Fats	Vitamins	Minerals	Fibre
Fruit Pulp	6g	65g	2g	A, C, D, E, B1, B2	Ca, K, P, Fe, Mg, Mn	10–12g
Fermented Seeds	25–35g	30–40g	15g	B1, B2, B3	K, Ca, Mg, Fe, P, Mn, Zn	4–8g

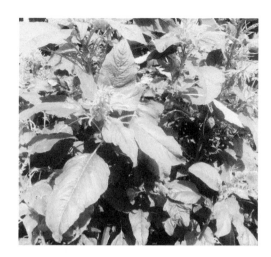

Amaranth

Local Names: *Callaloo; Calalou; Bledo; Uray; Efo; Madze; Imbuya; Boroboro; African Spinach*

Botanical Information: *Amaranthus spp (Amaranthaceae)*

Amaranth is an annual plant that originated in the Americas and is now widely distributed across the tropical world. There are many varieties of the plant developed in various parts of the world. Amaranth is regarded primarily as a green leafy vegetable, with a long history of culinary uses. In some varieties, the 'flowers' are well developed, bearing numerous, small seeds, which are used as a grain. The stems and leaves can vary from green to deep red or purple. The plant can tolerate a wide range of soil types but needs to have regular water and thrives best in temperatures from 20–40°C.

The seeds, which are abundant, germinate readily, and the plants can produce leaves within a month and continue to produce new leaves for a few months until replanting is necessary. Amaranth can therefore provide good quality leaves and stems which are nutritious and can be prepared in any number of ways.

Each year, across Africa, Asia and the Americas, hundreds of thousands of tonnes of amaranth are produced and form an important part of the diet for many millions of people. Despite this, amaranth is rarely mentioned in either books or documents about food and nutrition security. Given the fact that some varieties produce pseudo-grains, which are also nutritious, amaranth needs to be given a more prominent role in food security initiatives.

Food Products

The leaves and stems of the amaranth are the most widely used parts of the plant, and these do not require extensive cooking if they are picked when tender. More nutrients, especially vitamin C, are retained when the leaves are not cooked for long. The leaves have a pleasant taste and can be added to soups, stews, cooked alone or with fish and meat dishes. Amaranth leaves are rich in protein, with high levels of the key amino acid, lysine, and are comparable to spinach in terms of nutrients.

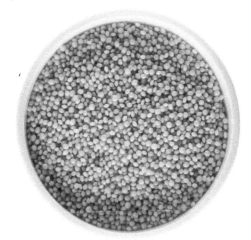

AMARANTH SEEDS

Amaranth seeds are small but plentiful and can be milled after parching. The flour produced is used to make flatbreads and pancakes and is rich in protein, B vitamins, and various minerals. The gluten-free flour can be mixed with wheat or other flour to make nutritious products.

History/Lore

Amaranth has been cultivated for more than 5,000 years in Central America and was one of the most important crops in Aztec culture. Grown primarily for its grains/seeds, revenues in the Aztec kingdom were often collected in amaranth, such was its value. The grain also played an essential role in their festivities and rituals. With the arrival of the Spanish colonialists, Aztec culture was deemed unchristian, and anything that seemed to be of importance to the people became a target for their anti-indigenous campaigns.

Soon amaranth was outlawed, and growing or being in possession of the grain or plant was severely punished. Despite the best efforts of Cortes and his invaders, which included the burning of amaranth fields, amaranth survived: more than 500 years later, amaranth in all its forms has made a comeback, both in its traditional homeland and as far away as Asia. Amaranth is taken from the Greek *amaranton*, which means 'ever living'. The plant has lived up to its name so far, without much support or fanfare, and millions of people continue to enjoy it and benefit from its nutrients.

Nutrition Information

Part of Plant	Protein	Carbohydrates	Fats	Vitamins	Minerals	Fibre
Leaves	2–3g	5g	2g>	A, C, K, B2, B6, B9	Ca, K, Fe, Zn, Mg, Se,	2g
Grain	12–15g	65g	2g	B1, B2, B3, B6, B9	Fe, Ca, Mg, K, Zn	2g

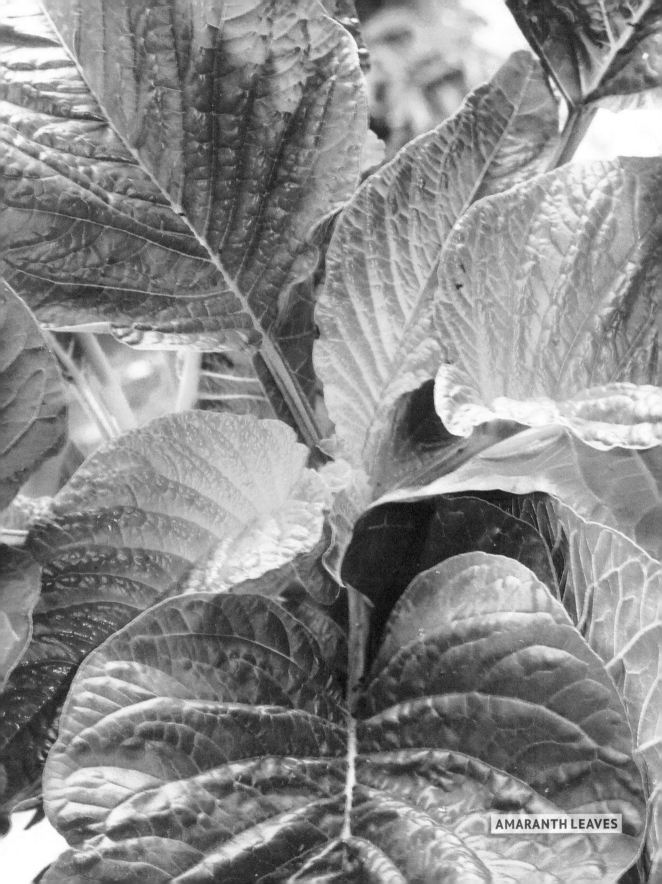

AMARANTH LEAVES

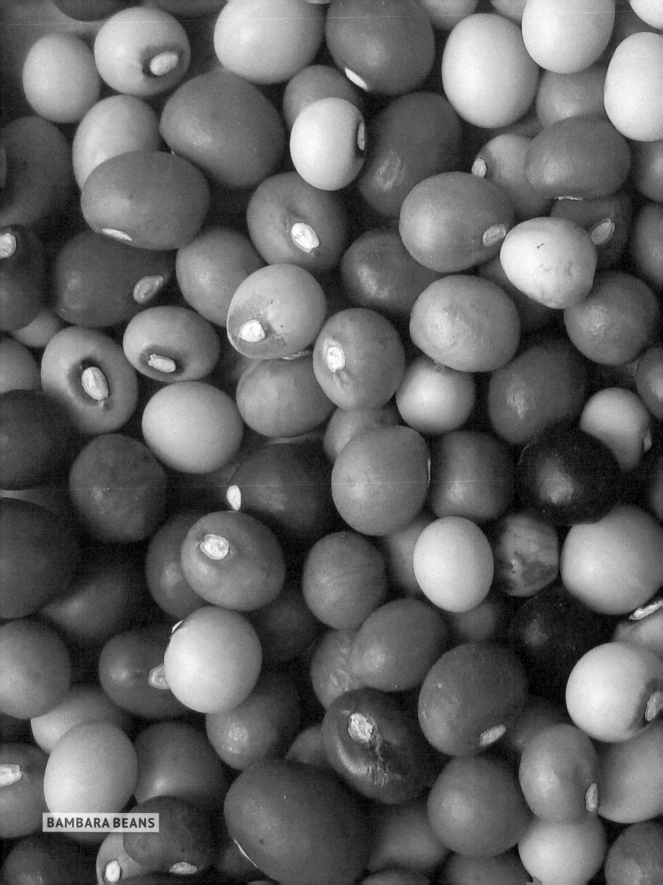

BAMBARA BEANS

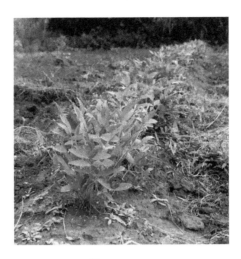

Bambara Bean

Local Names: *Bambara Groundnut; Earth Bean; Congo Goober; Voandzou; Souma; Pois Arachide; Mandubi d'Angola; Ababoi; Epi Roro; Gurjiya; Jugo; Njugu Bean; Nyimo; Thua Rang*

Botanical Information: *Vigna subterranea (Leguminosea/ Fabacea)*

Bambara bean is thought to have originated in what is today central Mali, but there are also those who believe it came from the area between northeastern Nigeria and Cameroon. The crop is now widely grown across the Sahel region as well as in parts of east and southern Africa. Bambara beans are grown in Brazil, where they are called *mandubi d'Angola*, and also in other South and Central American countries to a lesser extent. Bambara beans are now produced in significant quantity in Thailand, Malaysia and other parts of Southeast Asia and Oceania.

This annual plant can be erect and bushy or trailing, with creeping stems at ground level. Although called a bean, it actually bears underground, similar to groundnuts. The leaves are compound, made up of three leaflets, and the yellow flowers bear near the ground. Once the flowers have been pollinated, they send down a root-like tendril that goes below the ground in order to produce the beans or nuts. The beans reach maturity within 40 days after fertilisation, and each pod contains one or two beans, but there are types that bear three.

The pods are larger and rounder than that of the peanut, and the beans or nuts inside are about 1–1.5 cms. These are usually harvested when they are still quite immature: those that are picked when dry are very tough. Bambara beans come in a variety of colours from cream through red, purple and black or a combination of colours and patterns.

Bambara bean is considered the most drought-resistant of all the legumes but can thrive where there is significant rainfall, as long as rainfall is not heavy when the plant is flowering. Cultivation of Bambara beans was reduced in some areas of traditional production and displaced in many instances by groundnut. However, as climate change takes hold and experts recommend the use of low-input, sustainable crops, Bambara beans are seeing increased interest and research into its ability to provide reasonable yields in conditions where other crops struggle to survive.

Food Products

Bambara beans are related to both cow peas (*Vigna unguiculata*) and peanut or groundnut (*Arachis hypogaea*), and like these family members, the beans or nuts have high levels of essential amino acids and other key nutrients. It is rich in protein, has good quality carbohydrates and fats, and a high fibre content. Add to this the many vitamins and minerals in Bambara beans and it is easy to see how they can contribute to improved nutrition and health.

Immature Bambara beans are usually eaten boiled or roasted wherever they are grown. They are also combined with other grains such as maize or millet to make a soup or with groundnut to make a snack or soup.

The dried beans are usually de-hulled and pounded or ground into a flour that is used either alone or with other cereals to make a nutritious stiff porridge, similar to ugali or pap.

Preparation of the dry beans varies by area, country, culture and preference, but there are many dishes in which they are used. Dried beans are best soaked overnight before boiling and removing the seedcoat. It is then cooked either alone, added to stews or crushed, seasoned with spices and herbs and fried in either palm oil or shea butter. The flavour and texture of the de-hulled beans are similar to chickpeas or common beans.

Bambara bean flour can be mixed with wheat flour or others to make tasty baked products including bread. Good-quality plant milk can be extracted from Bambara beans similar to soya milk, and it has performed well in blind tests for taste and texture.

Medicinal Properties

Bambara beans provide such a well-balanced range of macro- and micronutrients that it can make a significant contribution to overall health improvement. Further, the high levels of fibre in the bean can contribute to reducing colon problems, help people living with diabetes to manage their condition and help with weight control.

In parts of West Africa, pregnant women slowly chew and swallow immature Bambara beans to reduce the nausea associated with morning sickness.

History/Lore

There has been a lot of debate as to where in Africa Bambara beans originated. The common name of the plant would suggest that it relates to the ethnic group called the Bambara or the area they occupy in what is now Mali. Plant geneticists have reported that the bean is most likely to have been first domesticated in the region, extending from the Jos Plateau in Nigeria to Garoua in Cameroon. These scientists have concluded this due to the wild beans that still grow in that region and the many types of domesticated Bambara beans that are cultivated there.

Bambara bean was first recorded in global botany in 1763, when it was given the name *Glycine subterranea*. While the *subterranea* part of the name has been consistent, the first name has been through a few changes. In 1806, a French botanist, working in Madagascar, adapted the local name for the plant from *voanjo* to *voandzou*, which is still the main French word for the plant.

As a result, the bean was then given the botanical name *Voandzeia subterranea*, which it kept until 1980, when it was concluded that the plant should be included in the same species as cow peas (*Vigna unguiculata*) and it was renamed *Vigna subterranea*. It has numerous common (local) names, but none seem to reflect its origins accurately, so we call it anything but where it originated, Congo goober, Mandubi d'Angola, Bambara bean.

Bambara beans are one of the crops from Africa that were cultivated by the various Maroon communities in Guyana, French Guyana and Suriname. There are records of these beans being used, up until recently, as much as or more than groundnuts; however, Bambara beans are not currently being as widely cultivated there as before.

Nutrition Information

Part of Plant	Protein	Carbohydrates	Fats	Vitamins	Minerals	Fibre
Beans	18–20g	50–60g	6.5%	A, E, B1, B2, B3	Fe, Ca, P, K, Mg, Zn,	5g

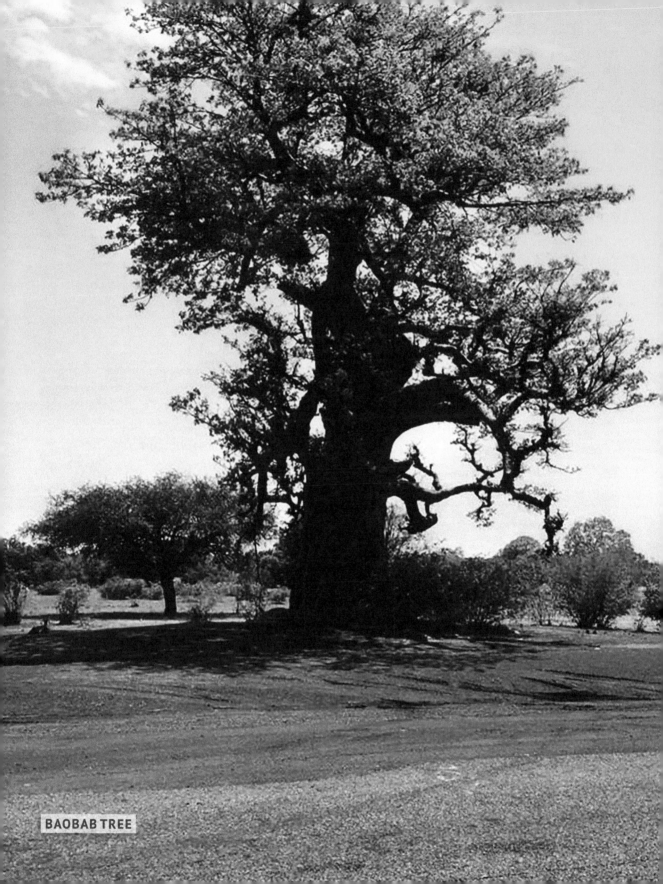

BAOBAB TREE

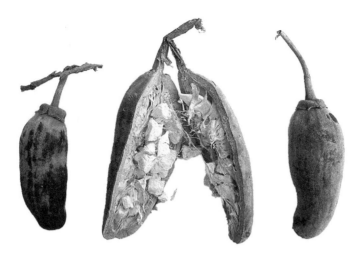

Baobab

Local Names: *Bui; Pain de singe; Mbuyu; Buhibab; Twege; Bokki; Odadie; Isimuhu; Sito; Hiru; Sira; Kuka; Odadie; Luru; Guinea Tamarind; Mapou Africain; Pan de manos; Monkey Tamarind; Sour Gourd; Dead Rat Tree; Jamaican Tamarind; Mapou Zombi*

Botanical Information: *Adansonia digitata (Malvaceae)*

Baobab is a tall, many-branched tree that can grow to a height of 25 metres, with a diameter ranging from 2–10 metres. This unique tree has been called 'a wonder of nature' due to its peculiar shape and many of its characteristics. The trunk is usually cylindrical but can taper towards the crown of the tree.

Baobab is widely distributed across savannah lands in the arid and semi-arid parts of Africa, from Senegal to Uganda and down through to South Africa. There are said to be eight types of the Adansonia species, one of which grows on mainland Africa, with a further six

on the island of Madagascar and another that grows in Australia. Baobab trees have been planted in India and other parts of South and Southeast Asia but do not occur on the same scale as trees in Africa. There are also baobab trees in the Caribbean, but they are not widely distributed there.

The tree can tolerate high temperatures and poor soils and is reputed to live for hundreds of years. The baobab tree is without leaves for eight months of the year: the leaves look like fingers of a hand and usually appear shortly before the rainy season. The large showy, white flowers only bloom at night and are a favourite of bats, which pollinate them. The flowers, which are beautiful with a fragrant odour, quickly fall and rot with an unpleasant odour.

Baobab trees grow quite slowly, with fruiting occurring from 8–23 years, with an average of 15–17 years, but considering that the lifespan of the tree is numbered in hundreds of years, this is not an unreasonable timespan. The fruit looks like a large, oval capsule; some have described it as looking like a rugby ball. The hard-shelled fruit is 20–30 cms long and up to 10 cms wide and hangs singly on a long stalk. The pod contains many seeds covered with a white powder, held together with fibrous strands running the length of the fruit. Once mature, the baobab tree can bear hundreds of fruits each season.

The tree is known by many different local names, but wherever it grows, it is regarded as having multipurpose uses as a source of food, medicine, shelter, fibre for making various products, wood for fuel and environmental regeneration.

Food Products

Young, tender baobab leaves are harvested during the rainy season and cooked fresh, but before the dry season arrives, the leaves are collected and dried for later use. The powdered leaves, which have their own names in different countries and cultures in Sub-Saharan Africa, are used in a variety of traditional dishes, especially in rural areas, providing a nutritious food source, particularly at times when other foods are scarce.

One theme that has emerged about the nutrients in the leaves, fruit pulp and seeds of the baobab is the variation in the amount of minerals and vitamins from different trees. Some of this could be due to soil and climatic condition, differences in the particular variety of the trees or the collection, storage and handling of the samples.

An analysis of dried baobab leaves for beta-carotene, carried out by Hoffman-La Roche of Switzerland, showed that the highest level was found in small leaves from young trees, which are shade dried. There are variations in the nutritional profile of the leaves depending on type of tree and local climatic conditions as well as method of drying.

Dried baobab leaves contain good-quality protein with five of eight essential amino acids and also have vitamins B2 and C, with high levels of calcium, manganese, zinc and, importantly, iron. The level of iron is said to be higher than from many other wild-gathered foods, which is important given the high rates of iron deficiency in populations who live in the savannah regions where baobab grows.

The fruit pulp is perhaps the most widely consumed part of the baobab tree, as it is eaten raw straight from the pod/shell, mixed with either hot or cold water or milk or with some form of grain porridge. Baobab fruit pulp is floury in texture with a slightly acidic taste that makes it a very versatile addition to all kinds of foods and beverages. The fruit pulp contains some protein, sugars and almost no fat, and has high levels of vitamin C and some B vitamins. Baobab fruit is also rich in a number of minerals such as iron, calcium, magnesium, zinc and phosphorous.

Baobab seeds are a nutritional powerhouse, containing protein, fats and high levels of minerals, including iron, calcium and zinc.

A high-quality oil is also extracted from the seeds, which has been found to be rich in mono- and polyunsaturated fatty acids. The beta-carotene content of baobab seed oil is twice that of palm oil and seven times that of corn oil.

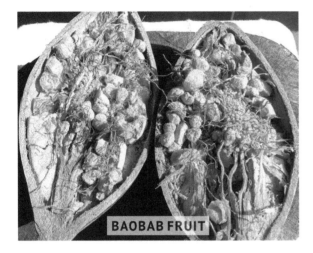
BAOBAB FRUIT

Medicinal Properties

There is a long tradition of using different parts of the baobab tree for medicinal purposes wherever it grows. The most common, widespread use is of the bark and fruit pulp to treat and prevent fevers, especially in cases of malaria and in some parts of Sub-Saharan Africa, the bark is regarded as a substitute for quinine.

Powdered leaves, fruit pulp, seeds and bark can be applied as a poultice to treat swellings, pain and for different kinds of wounds and skin infections. Baobab bark was exported in the past to Europe, as a treatment for fever and was traded as *cortex cael cedra*.

Antioxidants play a crucial role in preventing diseases such as cancer, cardiovascular disease and degenerative conditions, and baobab is rich in these substances.

Other Uses

Baobab has many other uses, of special interest is the tree's capacity to store significant amount of water, with estimates ranging from 200–4,000 gallons, depending on the size of the tree. It has been reported that if the trunk is kept well closed, the water can remain sweet for years. There is ongoing interest and research into the properties within the tree's structure and chemistry that helps the water to resist microbial contamination.

The inner bark of the tree and the root bark are sources of fibre that can be used to make, among other things, rope, baskets and fishing lines. The roots and green bark also produce dyes used in decoration. The hard fruit shells are used for fuel and increasingly to make decorative items, such as accessories and jewellery. The leaves, fruit shells and seedcake are used as fodder for livestock as well.

Baobab trees provide food and shelter for not just humans but many life forms: insects, birds and many large mammals including elephants.

Due to the antioxidant properties in baobab fruit pulp, increasing use is being made of pulp extracts that can extend the shelf life of other foods, beverages and cosmetic products as a natural preservative.

History/Lore

The baobab is one of the most iconic trees on the African savannah; its strange appearance and even stranger fruits are the stuff of legends and myths. Wherever the tree grows, there are tales about it and how it got its upside-down look, with its branches reaching into the air like roots. Most agree that it ended up this way as some kind of punishment or misfortune but with the assurance that it would at least become one of the most useful of all the trees.

Across Sub-Saharan Africa, baobab trees were used as a meeting and gathering place, and it was thought that when the elders were discussing important matters, they would get spiritual guidance from the tree. In some communities, the trees were used for burials. Baobab trees are widespread in areas where the slave trade routes passed and have borne witness to that inhuman enterprise. As most trees live for many hundreds of years, some, like the largest one in the centre of Saakpuli, in Northern Ghana, were used as a marketplace for trading enslaved people. Other large baobab trees were used as rest stops on the terrible march to the coast.

Baobab also made the journey across the Atlantic Ocean, and some of these trees survive in the Western Hemisphere to this day. The trees have been regarded as a useful but curious exotic shade tree in places like Florida and on some of the Caribbean islands. Trees have been either intentionally or accidentally cut down as being 'useless' due to lost traditional knowledge or were unable to survive the frequent hurricanes they may have encountered annually. Hurricanes are not a climatic feature where baobab originated, and they are not well suited to such severe winds.

There are still baobab trees in islands such as Barbados, Antigua, and Puerto Rico, and records show a few notable ones were in Kingston and St Elizabeth, Jamaica in the late 20th century, but their current status is not known. It has been reported that there are still a few trees in Haiti. The baobab tree is part of the Voodun or Voodoo tradition and as such still has religious and cultural significance, but with increased deforestation on the island, it could be under threat there.

St Croix in the US Virgin Islands has more than 100 trees – more than any other island in the Caribbean – including the most notable of all, the baobab tree in Grove Place. This tree is estimated to be 250–300 years old and was grown from seeds brought by an enslaved African, who planted it when he landed in St Croix. The tree was the focal point for historical social protest, and in 1878, during the infamous Fireburn Labour Riots, twelve women who were deemed to be ringleaders were burnt alive under the shadow of this baobab tree.

On St Thomas, Virgin Islands, where the tree also grows, the baobab is called Guinea Tamarind, due to the tart taste and is used to make beverages. It is thought that the person who planted the seeds came to these islands from the Guinea region of West Africa.

Nutrition Information

Part of Plant	Protein	Carbohydrates	Fats	Vitamins	Minerals	Fibre
Fruit Pulp	2–3g	65–80g	1g>	C, B3, B6	Ca, K, Fe, Mg, Zn	5–8g
Leaves	13–15g	60–70g	4–6g	A, C, B2	Ca, Fe, Mg, Zn	10–12g
Seeds	15–30g	40–60g	20–30g	A, B1, E	Fe, Ca, K, P, Mg, Zn	10–20g

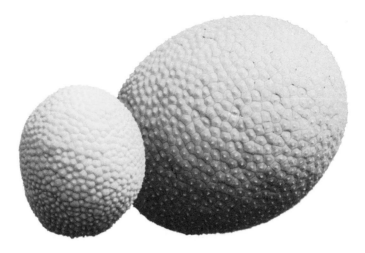

Breadfruit

Local Names: *Fruta de Pan; Fruit a Pain; Fruta Pao; Broodboom; Mazapan; Panapen; Rimas; Ulu*

Botanical Information: *Artocarpus altilis (Moraceae)*

Breadfruit is thought to have originated in Western Pacific islands such as New Guinea and the Maluku Islands. Botanists are still unsure as to whether the seedless variety (*Artocarpus altilis*) evolved from the seeded type (*Artocarpus camansi*) or is a separate sub-species. There are now a number of varieties of both seeded and seedless breadfruit across the tropical world. To ensure that there is little confusion in this book, the seedless varieties will be included under 'Breadfruit' and the seeded type will be referred to as 'Breadnut'.

The breadfruit tree is a large evergreen, which can grow to a height of 30 metres and has many spreading branches, with large, lobed leaves, 15–60 cms long. The tree bears both male and female flowers, and the fruit produced can have an oblong, oval or round shape. The texture of the skin of the fruit ranges from smooth to spiny depending on the variety. They are green when immature and gradually become yellow when ripe.

Breadfruit grows best in humid, tropical lowlands, but some varieties can be tolerant of other climatic conditions. The tree thrives in temperatures ranging from 20–35°C with 2–3,000 mm annual rainfall. When immature, the fruit is hard and the flesh is white to cream-coloured and starchy, becoming softer and more pungent as it ripens. When cut, all parts of the tree including the fruit have a milky, sticky latex.

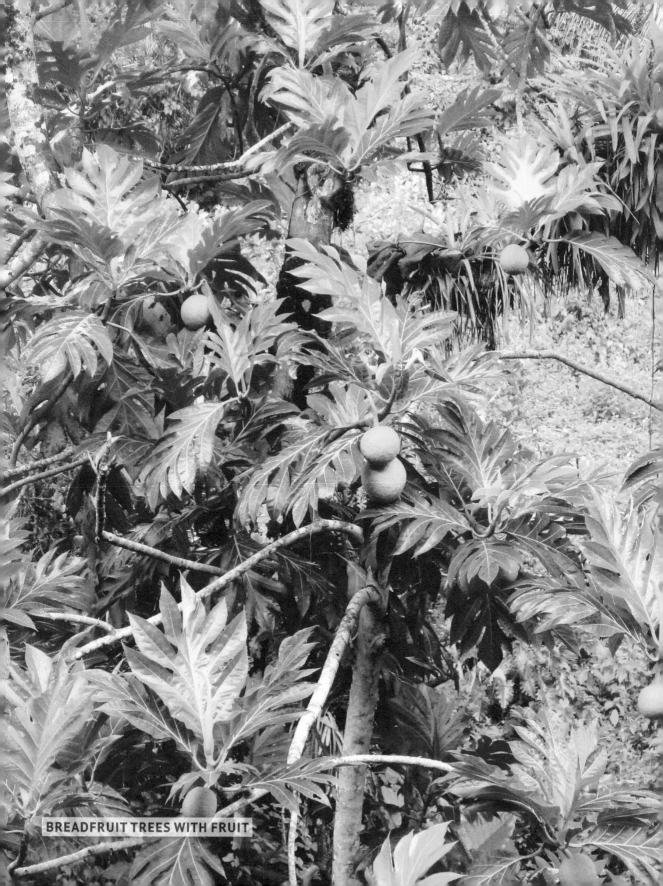

BREADFRUIT TREES WITH FRUIT

Globally, breadfruit production is highest in the Caribbean and Pacific regions, but there is significant production in parts of Asia and Africa. Breadfruit can be found from Southern Senegal to South-West Cameroon across the Congo Basin through Uganda and down to Mozambique. It is thought that both varieties of breadfruit first arrived in Africa via Ghana as a result of missionaries who had been in the Caribbean and thought that the plant could be beneficial to the local populations.

Food Products

Breadfruit is a very versatile food and can be used at almost all stages of its development. The immature fruit is used like a root vegetable, such as potato, so can be boiled, roasted, fried, steamed or added to stews, salads and soups. In many Pacific islands, breadfruit is roasted on an open fire or in traditional, underground ovens on preheated stones. The ripe breadfruit, which gets sweeter as it matures, is also versatile and can be prepared in different ways. It can be roasted or steamed like the immature ones or it can be used to make cakes, puddings and other desserts and fried as chips.

Apart from breadfruit's versatility, it also has a lot to offer in terms of nutrition, especially when compared to other common starchy root vegetables. It has more protein than taro, potato or even white rice; in fact, breadfruit has higher amounts of vitamins, carbohydrates and minerals except for phosphorous and potassium.

In some countries, thin slices of unripe breadfruit are dried and pounded to make flour, which can be mixed with wheat flour to make a wide range of baked products.

For people living with conditions that make them gluten intolerant, breadfruit flour can be mixed with coconut oil and used as a gluten-free pizza base.

The male flower is scraped, boiled and diced before being stewed in syrup and sometimes even coloured and used as part of dried-fruit mix in baking.

Medicinal Properties

Raw ripe breadfruit can be purgative, and even the cooked unripe fruits can help with bowel health as it is high in fibre.

A decoction of breadfruit leaves is used across the Caribbean to treat high blood pressure, liver problems and also for relieving asthma.

Other Uses

Breadfruit leaves are eaten by animals such as goats and the wood used in light construction and for making furniture. The wood is also used to make traditional Hawaiian drums. The dried male 'sword' is burnt as an insect repellent.

History/ Lore

Europeans are said to have come across breadfruit in the late 16th century in the Marquesas Islands in the Pacific. Although stories of these trees bearing starchy fruits circulated from time to time, it was not until the late 18th century and following a number of famines in the Caribbean islands, that colonial powers such as France, Spain and Britain began to explore the fruit's potential to feed enslaved people in their colonies.

The British effort to take breadfruit plants from Tahiti to the Caribbean by Captain Bligh in 1787 became the stuff of legends when the mission was thwarted by a mutiny on his ship, the *Bounty*. Finally, in 1793 on his second journey, Captain Bligh brought five different varieties – over 200 breadfruit plants – to Jamaica. Bligh had left breadfruit trees in the British colony of St Kitts before his arrival in Jamaica. Both seeded and seedless trees flourished on the island and other British-ruled islands, and even in the 21st century, Jamaica remains one of the largest producers of *A. altilis*.

In many cultures, breadfruit trees are symbolic of bounty and perseverance through adversity, and there is a majesty and resilience in the characteristics of the tree. These virtues have been observed and captured in different cultures in various ways. In Jamaica, there is a proverb that says 'The more you chop the breadfruit root, the more it springs'. The future trees usually spring from cuts along the large root system, so what should be injurious is actually life-giving.

Nutrition Information

Part of Plant	Protein	Carbohydrates	Fats	Vitamins	Minerals	Fibre
Fruit	3–5g	30–50g	1g>	C, B1, B2, B3, B5, B6, B9	K, P, Mg, Fe, Ca	5g

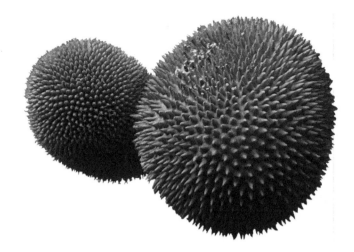

Breadnut

Local Names: *Breadfruit Nut; Chataignier; Chataine; Castana; Kamansi; Pana de Pepitas; Kapiak;*

Botanical Information: *Artocarpus camansi (Moraceae)*

Breadnut (*A. camansi*) is thought to have originated in New Guinea, and islands such as the Philippines were said to be the source of the trees that were taken by the Spanish colonisers to Central and South America and the Caribbean. Later, the French also transported both varieties to their colonies in the New World. Breadnut is not as widely grown in Pacific islands such as Hawaii and Tahiti, where breadfruit is a very important staple.

There is another tropical tree called 'breadnut', but this is a completely different species (*Brosimum alicastrum*) known in Central America as Maya Nut or Ramon Nut.

The breadnut tree is similar in most of its characteristics to that of the breadfruit (*A. altilis*), described above. The trees are distributed by birds, bats and other mammals that feed on the flesh and drop the large seeds. The fruit is almost oblong, 15–20 cms long, weighing between 500–800 grams, its skin ranging in colour from green to yellow-green with a soft spiny texture.

Compared to breadfruit, there is little flesh in the fruit of the breadnut, and they are grown mainly for the seeds. The flesh, which can range from white to pale yellow in colour, becomes softer and sweeter as the fruit matures. The number of seeds in a fruit can vary as can the size, but they usually have a soft, light-brown seedcoat, which means they can sprout very quickly, sometimes even while in the fallen fruit. The seeds make up 30–50% of the total weight of the breadnut.

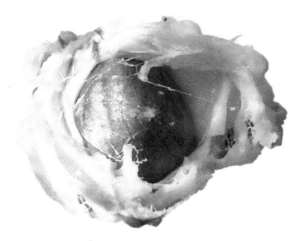

BREADNUT SEED

Food Products

In many countries, the immature breadnut is sliced thinly and prepared in different ways. The sliced fruit is used like a starchy vegetable and can be cooked by itself or added to stews and soups; however, the seed or nut is the main part used. This nutritious nut is a good source of protein and is also high in carbohydrates, fibre and key vitamins and minerals. The seed provides good fatty acids and can produce a useful plant-based oil, that smells like peanut oil, with properties that are similar to olive oil.

The dried breadnut is sometimes ground into a flour that can be mixed with other flours to make a nutritious composite product with many applications, including baked goods, porridges and functional food products.

Many people liken the taste of breadnut to chestnuts, and there should be a lot of scope for commercial processing of this under-used seed. The seeds can be roasted, boiled and tinned or made into nut butter. There is also the potential to make a milk substitute from the seed, either by itself or as part of a blend with other nuts or seeds.

Medicinal Properties

The high levels of nutrients in the breadnut can contribute to overall health improvement as part of healthy diet. Various parts of the tree are used traditionally for medicinal purposes. The breadnut leaves are used for hypertension and asthma as well as skin conditions. A decoction of the bark is also taken in Southeast Asia for stomach problems, including dysentery.

Other Uses

The breadnut tree, as stated above, is similar in many respects to the breadfruit tree and shares many properties. The timber is also used for fuel and to carve craft items; the latex in various parts of the tree is useful as a caulk or as bird lime. The dried male flowers are burned and used as an insect repellent.

Nutrition Information

Part of Plant	Protein	Carbohydrates	Fats	Vitamins	Minerals	Fibre
Seed	15–20g	50–70g	5–7g	A, E, B3, B5, B6, B9	Ca, P, K, Fe, Mg	3g

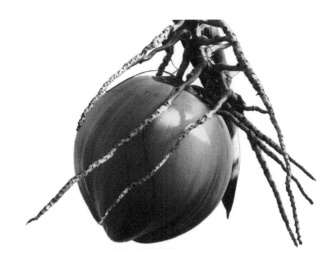

Coconut

Local Names: *Coconut Palm; Palma de Coco; Cocos, Noix de Coco; Cocoyer; Nyior; Naral; Nyiog*

Botanical Information: *Cocos nucifera (Arecaceae)*

Coconut is a tall, slender tree without branches that has a crown of 20–40 large pinnate leaves, ranging from 4–6 metres long. It has been called one of the ten most useful trees in the world, as reflected in its Sanskrit name, *kalpavriksha*, which means 'tree that gives everything that is needed'; this term is also used in relation to any reference to a mythical, wish-fulfilling tree.

There are many theories about the origins of the coconut, but it is generally agreed that it is native to the region around Indonesia, the Philippines and South India. The plant has been distributed widely by marine and human movements and now grows in almost 100 countries globally. Countries such as Sri Lanka, Philippines and New Guinea are among the leading producers of the coconut, but increasing demand, locally and internationally, means that there needs to be further increase in the cultivation of coconuts, wherever they grow.

Coconuts are divided into two main types, the 'tall' and the 'dwarf', with any number of hybrids from them, each type having some kind of distinguishing characteristic related to size, quality or the maturity cycle. The tall can reach up to 30 metres in height, while the dwarf is rarely more than 10 metres high. The tall grows more slowly and does not fruit until 8–10 years after planting, but the tree will continue to produce fruit monthly for 40–90

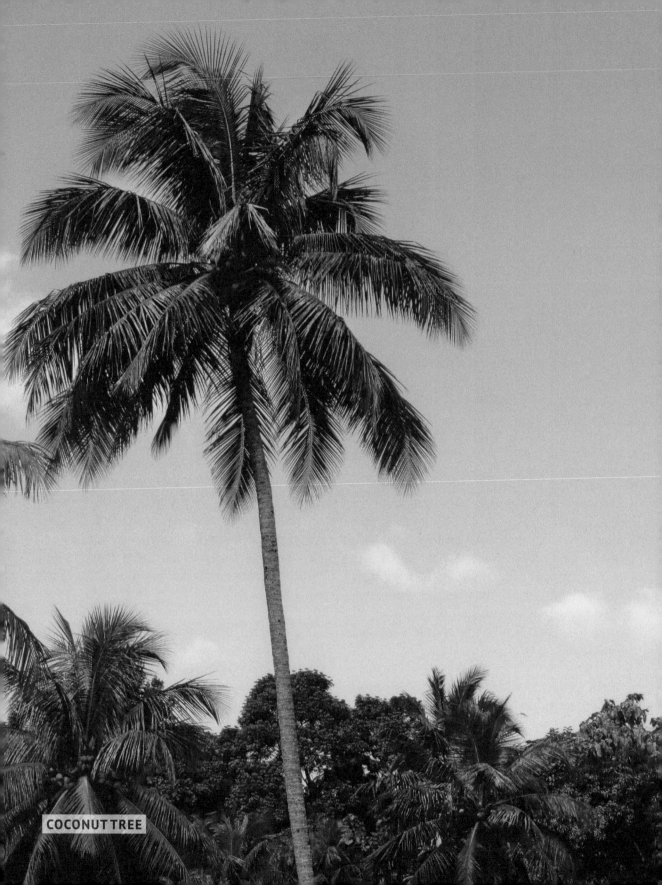

COCONUT TREE

years. The dwarf trees fruit within five years, but only live for 30–40 years. Coconut trees flower and fruit all year round, and the cycle from flowering to maturity takes 12 months.

Both male and female flowers are borne in a tough double sheath called a spathe. As the spathe opens wider, the female flowers develop into the fruit that we call a coconut, which is not classified as a nut but as a fibrous drupe. When the spathe dries and falls away, bunches of up to 30 coconuts develop over the course of 9–12 months. The colour of the outer skin of the fruit can be yellow, green or orange but becomes brown as it matures and dries.

The outer 'husk' is made up of a brown, dense fibre, known as 'coir', which encloses the seed of the fruit, the 'nut'. The outer shell of this nut gets browner and harder as the fruit matures. Inside, it has a thin, brown rind covering white flesh that thickens and hardens with maturity (1–3 cm). The cavity of the seed contains up to 500 ml of liquid, commonly called coconut water, that lessens as the nut dries.

Coconuts tend to be cultivated on coastal plains, whether on sandy soil or clay, as long as it is well drained. The tree prefers good rainfall, but the dwarf variety is much more susceptible to drought than the tall type. The trees can tolerate not just salt spray but saline soils as well, generally being able to produce in a variety of climatic and geographic conditions. Due to the fact that the trees are usually planted quite far apart, it is possible to intercrop them with a wide range of plants.

Food Products

The coconut tree produces an amazing array of goods, edible and otherwise, as will be seen later. Once the tree produces its inflorescence, the stalk can be 'tapped' to obtain a sweet sap, which is underutilised, considering its nutritional profile. It has been estimated that up to 1.5 litres of sap can be tapped daily without serious effects on the quality and quantity of the fruits produced.

The sap, called *neera* or *tuba*, is either drunk fresh or left to ferment, which begins within hours if left without refrigeration. The fermented, alcoholic beverage is called toddy in parts of Asia, where it is widely consumed. The sap can also be boiled into a syrup or molasses, similar to maple syrup; when crystallised, this becomes coconut sugar, which is reported to have some health benefits.

Water from the immature fruits has always been popular wherever the tree grows but has now gained widespread international interest and is marketed as a healthy rehydrating fluid. The 'jelly-like' flesh in the immature fruit is eaten raw, but it is the flesh of the mature nuts that makes up the bulk of the international coconut trade.

Coconut flesh can be eaten raw but has many and varied culinary uses as coconut milk, desiccated coconut, coconut cream and oil. The oil is also used in the manufacture of margarine, desserts, baked goods and confectionery, including ice cream and milk-substitute products. The roots of the tree can be roasted, ground and used as a coffee substitute.

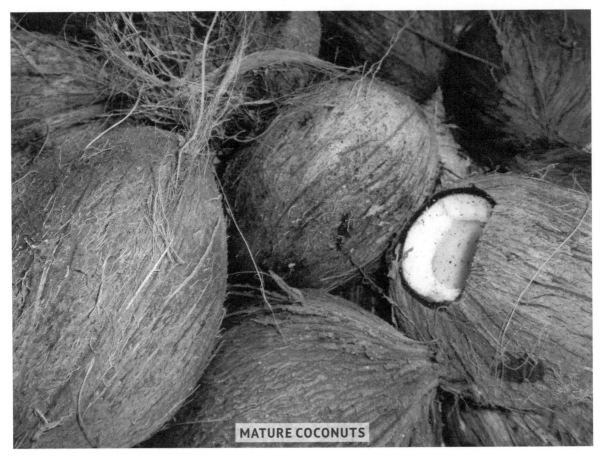

MATURE COCONUTS

Medicinal Properties

Almost all parts of the coconut tree and its produce are believed to have medicinal properties. Coconut water is reputed to reduce blood pressure due to the high levels of potassium and people living with type 2 diabetes can drink the water of very young coconuts, as it is low in sugar while providing useful trace minerals and electrolytes.

The high fibre of mature coconut meat helps to slow release of glucose in the blood. Coconut oil is mildly laxative and also has anti-inflammatory properties. In South Asia, it is traditionally mixed with turmeric and used to relieve sore joints and muscles.

When the dried nut is left to sprout, a spongy kernel is formed inside. This is sometimes eaten, but in the Pacific Islands, they are dried and used to treat diarrhoea and dysentery. The sap juice is taken by women to promote recovery after childbirth, and the roots of the tree are decocted and used for stomach and bladder disorders.

Other Uses

Coconut oil has long been cherished for its emollient properties for skin and hair and is used in the commercial manufacturing of soaps, detergents, candles, lubricants cosmetic and pharmaceutical products. The leaves are plaited and made into roof thatching and matting for walls and floors. All parts of the leaves can be made into various household items such as mats, baskets and brooms.

The coir, which is the dried fibrous inner mass that surrounds the nut, is used as stuffing for seats and mattresses as well as to make fibre. The shell of the nut is used to make utensils, jewellery, musical instruments and other craft items. A charcoal from the shells is used in some industrial processes, and the trunk wood is used for furniture, flooring and other purposes.

History/Lore

One of the many myths about coconuts concern the three eyes of the dried nut. In the countries where coconuts are native, there are stories that tell of these eyes looking like a monkey or an eel, depending on tradition. In fact, the word 'coco' is an old Portuguese word meaning head or skull: the sailors who first travelled to the Indian Ocean region and saw the dried coconut thought the three eyes made the nut look like a face.

The eyes are at the stem end of the coconut. One of them is soft, and beneath it is the embryo, which starts off the size of a pea and increases as the nut ages. If you need to get to the sweet water inside a dried nut, find the soft eye and drill in with a pointed implement.

Another myth relates to the so called 'Coconut Pearl', which is said to be found in the cavity of a 'blind' nut; this is one without eyes that has dried out naturally. The 'rare' pearl is said to be similar to aragonite or calcium carbonate. It is creamy white and smooth with faint patterning and when 'found' is used in jewellery, but more importantly, it is regarded as being a great omen for anyone who finds one. In some cultures, it represents good luck, wealth, purity and spirituality.

However, experts are sceptical of the authenticity of these 'pearls' and are convinced that they are not from a coconut. Gem specialists have stated that there is no possible mechanism by which something within the coconut can morph into such a dense material within the life cycle of the fruit. This has not stopped either the beliefs surrounding the coconut pearl or the profitable trade in these 'gems'.

Nutrition Information

Part of Plant	Protein	Carbohydrates	Fats	Vitamins	Minerals	Fibre
Mature Fruit	2–4g	15–20g	30–40g	C, E, B1, B3, B5, B6	K, P, Ca. Fe, Mn, Zn, Se	7–10g
Coconut Milk	2g	5g	20–25g	C, B1, B2, B3, B6	K, P, Ca, Fe, Zn, Mg	2–3g
Coconut Flour	10–15g	20–30g	10–15g	B1, B2, B3, B5, B6	K, Fe, Mg, P, Zn, Se	20g

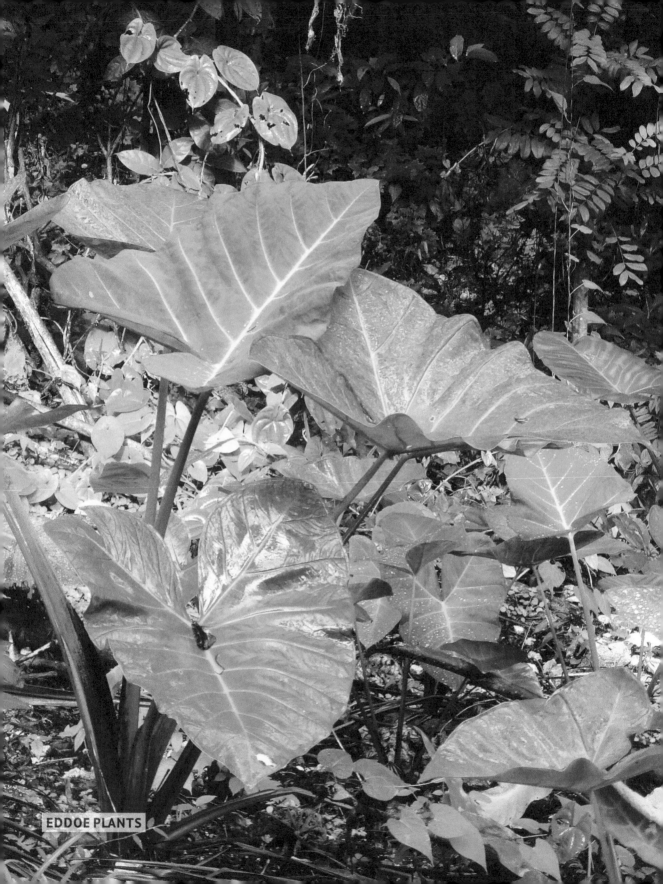

EDDOE PLANTS

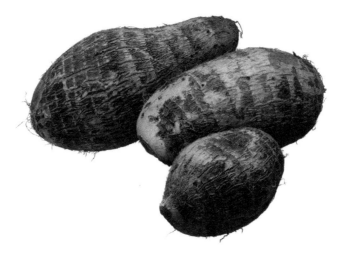

Cocoyam (Eddoe)

Local Names: *Tannia; Coco; Malanga; Tanier; Yautia; Chou Caraibe; Mangarita; Nampi, New Cocoyam*

Botanical Information: *Xanthasoma sagittifolium (Araceae)*

Cocoyam is the name given to two related species which are sometimes confused or seen as interchangeable. *Xanthasoma sagittifolium* and *Colcasia esculenta* share a number of characteristics (both belong to the wider *Araceae* family) but are different plants. For the purpose of this book, they will be referred to as Cocoyam (Eddoe) and Cocoyam (Taro).

Cocoyam (Eddoe) is said to have originated in the north-eastern regions of South America and was most likely spread by native peoples as they migrated across the Caribbean islands. Eddoe then reached West Africa by way of the transatlantic trade in enslaved peoples and now also grows in tropical parts of Asia and the Pacific.

Eddoe, unlike taro, prefers well-drained soil, tolerates more saline soils, can be grown in more upland areas and is able to tolerate less rainfall than taro. Similar in looks to taro, the main differences are that the stalks of the eddoe attach at the edge of the arrowhead-shaped leaves, unlike those of the taro, which attach at the centre.

Another significant difference between the plants is the way in which the tubers present. The taro usually has one main tuber, but the eddoe produces a number of tubers or corms of varying size and weight.

Food Products

The starch from eddoe is similar to that of taro, with high digestibility and different uses. There are more varieties of eddoes than taro, ranging in colour from pale white to pinkish-purple and the texture can be soft and mushy right through to firm and powdery, when cooked. Eddoe can be prepared in a number of ways: as a side dish, in soups and stews, or it can be baked, roasted or made into chips.

Eddoe can also be made into flour and used like fufu, mashed and added as a thickener to soups, or substituted for mashed potatoes. It is one of the tubers used in some recipes for traditional Jamaican puddings, and with its nutty flavour and many nutrients, it could be used to make various starchy and functional food products.

Flour made from eddoe tubers could be combined with grain or legume flour to make baked goods as well as a range of extruded products such as pasta and shaped snacks. The leaves of the eddoe and taro are used in similar ways and have similar nutrients and active compounds.

Medicinal Properties

Eddoe's digestible starches can be used as a weaning food for infants, as an alternative for those with impaired digestion, who are gluten intolerant or recovering after illness. The high fibre content of both tubers and leaves can help to improve digestive health and manage type 2 diabetes.

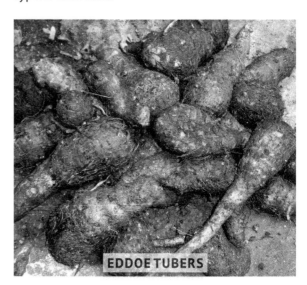

EDDOE TUBERS

Nutrition Information

Part of Plant	Protein	Carbohydrates	Fats	Vitamins	Minerals	Fibre
Corm/Tuber	2g	20g	1g>	A, C, B1, B2, B3, B5, B6	K, Fe, Mg, Zn, Ca, P, Mn	2g
Leaves	3g	5g	2g>	C, A	Fe, K, Ca, P	3g
Flour	3–4g	60g	2g	C, A, B	Fe, Ca, Zn, P, Mn	5–7g

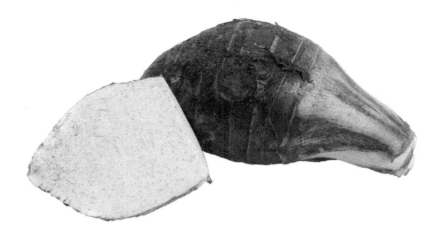

Cocoyam (Taro)

Local Names: *Dasheen; Old Cocoyam; Elephant Ear; Malanga; Taya; Arbi; Brobey*

Botanical Information: *Colocasia esculenta (Araceae)*

As mentioned earlier, there are two different root crops that are called cocoyam and which share many characteristics. Cocoyam (Taro) is thought to have originated in Southeast Asia or the Pacific region but is regarded as pan-tropical. It is now grown in Asia, Oceania, Central and South America, the Caribbean and Africa, mainly for its starchy tuber, but in many countries also for its leaves.

The plant grows from a whole tuber or a part of one, the long stems coming directly from the tuber, with large, heart-shaped leaves at the end of these stems. The leaves join the stem in the centre of the leaves, the spot often being seen as a round, purplish patch. Taro can reach a height of 1–2 metres, with leaves that can be up to 50 cms in length and vary in colour from green to purplish green. The tuber, which matures within 7–10 months of planting, can weigh up to 5 kg, depending on variety and type of soil it grows in.

The flesh of the taro ranges from white to purple, and there is evidence that those with coloured flesh contain other micronutrients or bioactive substances. Currently, both types of taro have declined in production and consumption compared to other tubers such as cassava, yam and sweet potato. Taro compares very favourably with these other root crops in terms of taste, nutrition and versatility.

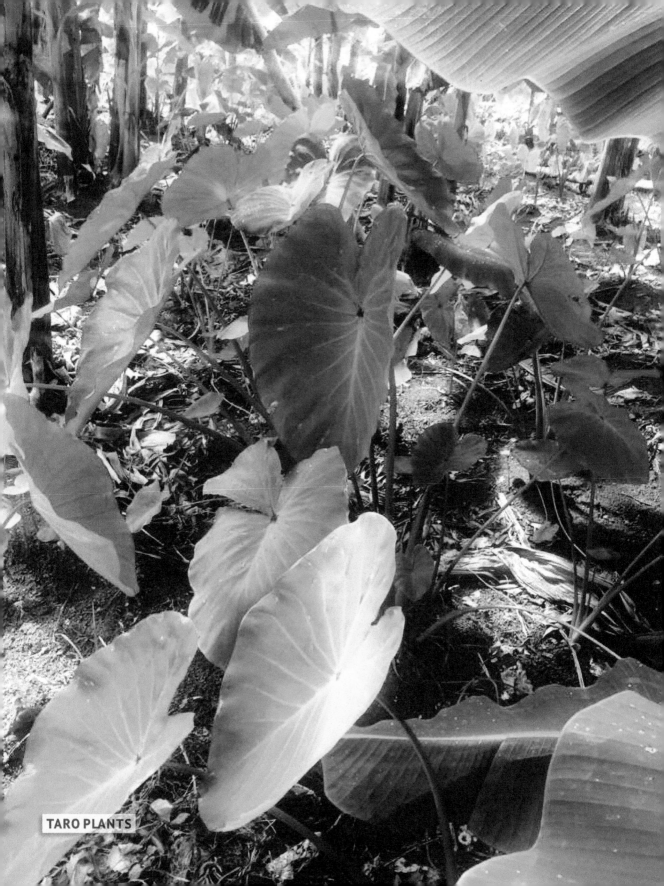

TARO PLANTS

Nigeria, Ivory Coast and Cameroon are the leading producers globally, with over 3.5 million tonnes annually produced in Nigeria alone. Asia and Oceania are also major producers, with China being second only to Nigeria, according to the most recent figures. There is, however, more room for increased cultivation, in light of the commercial potential of all parts of the plant.

Food Products

Wherever taro grows, it is used in various ways in very diverse diets, although not as much as it should be. The starchy tuber is the main edible part of the plant, but the leaves are very nutritious, and in some places, they are consumed as a vegetable in greater quantity than the tubers. Both leaves and tubers, however, can be toxic if eaten raw, due to high levels of oxalates in all parts of the plant.

The starch produced by taro has excellent digestibility, with high levels of mucilage. Like other root crops, taro can be boiled, baked, roasted, fried or dried. It is mashed and given to babies as a weaning food, either by itself or mixed with other tubers and vegetables. The taro flour is used to make fufu in Ghana and Nigeria and other parts of West Africa. It is added to soups, stews and porridges or made into beverages. The flour can also be combined with wheat, corn or other cereals to produce, nutritious blends for baked and other products. Taro and other tubers are grated, mixed with spices and coconut to make a delicious traditional pudding in Jamaica, and in Trinidad and Tobago, boiled taro is the base for a chilled punch.

Taro leaves can be blanched or boiled, depending on age of the leaf, before being cooked alone like spinach or added to other dishes. In Trinidad and Tobago, the heart-leaves are harvested and sold widely in bundles as 'calaloo', a name usually used for amaranth in other parts of the Caribbean. The heart-leaves are said to have lower levels of oxalates – the main reason for the plant's toxicity. In Hawaii and parts of Southeast Asia, the young leaves are cooked in coconut cream, with or without added spices. The leaves have good amounts of protein, are rich in vitamin A, C and E and minerals such as iron, magnesium and calcium.

Medicinal Properties

The high fibre in both leaves and tubers helps to regulate blood sugar levels and control insulin release, which is beneficial in the management of type 2 diabetes. Potassium is useful in the prevention and treatment of high blood pressure, all of which improves overall cardiovascular health.

Various parts of taro have been used in Ayurveda healing practice for centuries to treat health issues including liver problems, snake bites and other ailments. There is ongoing research in India and elsewhere into compounds extracted from taro leaf and stem extracts which are 'pharmacologically active'. The starch and gum from taro tubers have commercial application in the pharmaceutical industry. Taro flour and dried leaves could be processed to be utilised in different functional foods.

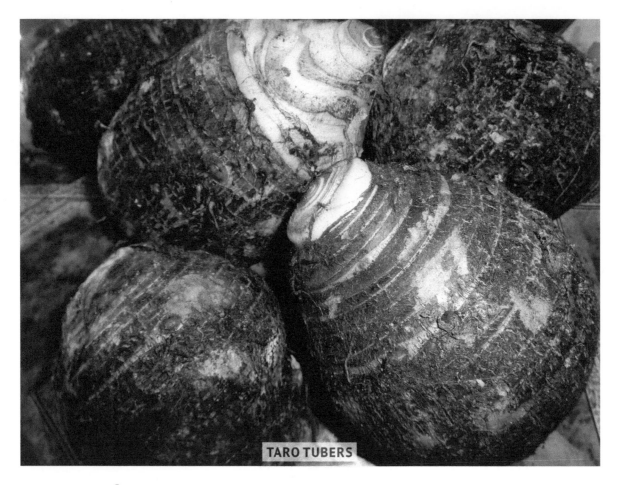

TARO TUBERS

Nutrition Information

Part of Plant	Protein	Carbohydrates	Fats	Vitamins	Minerals	Fibre
Tuber/Corm	1–2g	30g	1g>	A, C, E, B1, B2, B3, B5, B6, B9	Ca, Fe, Mg, Zn, K, P	4–7g
Leaves	5g	6g	1g>	A, C, B1, B2	Ca, K, Fe, Mn, P	3g
Flour	3–5g	70–75g	1g>	A, C, E, B	Ca, K, Fe, P, Zn	3–5g

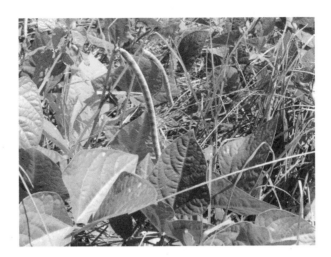

Cow Peas

Local Names: *Blackeye Peas; Niebe; Agwa; Akidiani; Barbata; Kunde; Field Bean; Nori; Boo; Chichara de Vaca; Southern Bean; Lupia; Karkala*

Botanical Information: *Vigna unguiculata (Leguminosae)*

The cow pea is one of the most widely planted native legumes in Sub-Saharan Africa, second only to the peanut in terms of area of farmland under production. It is the most economically important, indigenous African legume crop. The plant is said to have originated in the Sahel region of West Africa thousands of years ago, very near to the current main areas of production, and has evolved into the numerous varieties that now exist.

It is now grown from Senegal eastward to Somalia and southward to Botswana, Zimbabwe and Mozambique. Northern Nigeria and Niger are the main areas of production, with annual figures of 5 million tonnes of the

6.7 million tonnes produced in Africa. Despite the fact that cow peas are grown in more than 30 African countries, there still needs to be substantial increase in production. This would increase the crop's role in food and nutrition security in more countries outside of the current production centres in West Africa, especially in East and Southern Africa.

Cow peas are widely distributed across parts of Asia, Oceania, South America, the Caribbean and the south of the USA. It is believed that cow peas were brought to the New World by enslaved people, for whom this was an important and familiar food in their diet. It has

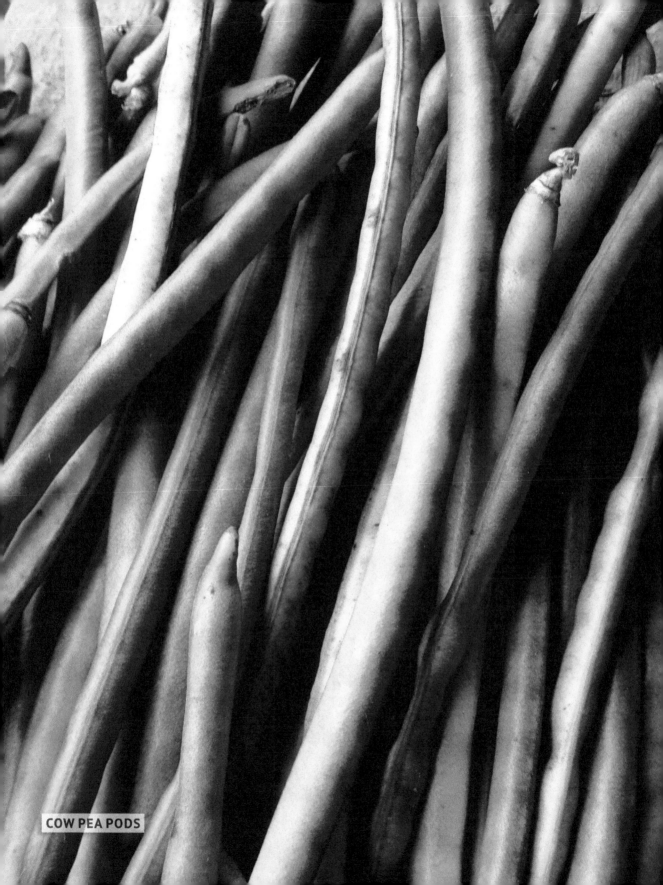

COW PEA PODS

been estimated that more than 200 million people consume this legume daily.

Cow pea is an annual crop with many varieties that range from those that are short, erect plants to those that are trailing and climbing ones (20–200 cms), depending on type and growing conditions. The flowers can range from white through pink and purple, and the peas themselves come in a whole host of colours from white, red, through to brown and black. The most common types are the white ones with the black dot in the middle, the typical 'black eye' that gives this bean one of its common names. The pods can bear from 8–20 peas, which are almost kidney shaped.

Due to the diversity of cow peas, the mature peas can be ready in anything from 60–240 days, depending on type and growing conditions. The plant grows in a wide variety of soils, helping to replenish any soil it grows in. Most varieties are drought-tolerant and can survive on less than 300 mm of rainfall annually but do less well in humid or wet environments. The crop can also thrive at relatively high elevation so long as it is planted during the hotter months.

Food Products

Cow peas are very nutritious, being rich in protein, carbohydrates, vitamins and minerals. The plant can be eaten at all stages of growth: the young leaves can be eaten as greens; the young pods can be eaten whole as a vegetable; the fresh and dried mature peas can be cooked alone or in combination with other grains and cereals.

Some of the most well-known and loved dishes from West Africa are made from cow peas in different forms. Akara is a delicious blend of boiled, mashed cow peas with lots of spices and fried into fritters. Moin-moin is from cow pea meal, seasoned with various spices made into balls and steamed. Waakye is a popular dish from the north of Ghana, made from rice and cow peas, with a distinctly red colour, and it made the long journey from that region to the Caribbean with the help of enslaved people. Rice and peas or beans as a dish is found in some form all over the Caribbean, although over time, the type of peas used may have changed. But there are many other dishes that include cow peas, combined with other legumes or grains such as maize or rice, and each region has their own speciality made from this versatile legume.

Considering the nutrition that cow peas deliver, it is a very under-rated and under-utilised food crop that needs more investment and research to address any challenges that inhibit this legume's potential.

Other Uses

Cow peas' deep roots help to stabilise soil, and the dense cover and shade that it offers helps to protect the ground and preserve moisture, all of which are useful characteristics in the dry regions where the legume grows. Cow peas are often planted with other crops which benefit from their soil-enriching properties. The plant also provides much-needed forage for livestock, often in areas with little else to graze on.

History/Lore

As noted earlier, cow peas reached the Americas during the time of slavery; it grew well in the south of the United States and was eaten by indigenous natives, European settlers and those of African descent for whom it was a beloved, traditional staple.

Over time, cow peas, blackeye peas, field beans or southern beans – as they were called locally – were mostly consumed by poorer people, who had long relied upon them, when

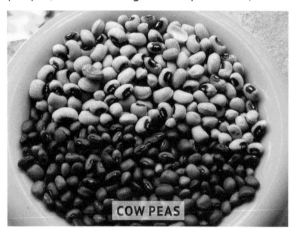

COW PEAS

other crops failed or had low yield. Cow peas became more popular as cattle fodder (hence the name), and there were thousands of acres of the peas growing almost wild in some parts of the South.

The American Civil War took a heavy toll on the Confederate states, and many plantations and farms were torched or had crops laid to waste as an added dimension of defeat. The humble cow peas were left because the Northern soldiers did not consider the crop as human food. Many people in the South turned to the cow peas after the war and found numerous ways to prepare them and help survive very difficult times.

Hoppin John is a traditional southern dish originated by enslaved Africans and is made from cow peas, rice, pork, hot pepper and other spices. Every New Year's Day, this humble bean of African origin is enjoyed by Southerners of all backgrounds as a symbol of good luck, having played such a crucial role in their post-civil-war survival.

Nutrition Information

Part of Plant	Protein	Carbohydrates	Fats	Vitamins	Minerals	Fibre
Immature Pods	3–5g	10g	2–3g	A, C, B1, B2, B3, B9	Ca, Fe, K	3g
Dried Peas	20–30g	60g	2–3g	B1, B2, B3, B5, B6, B9	Fe, Ca, K, Mn, P, Zn, Mg, Se	10–15g
Leaves	10–15g	1g>	3–4g	A, C, B1, B2, B3, B9	Fe, Ca, Zn, Mn, P, K, Mg	10–20g
Flour	20–25g	60g	2g>	B1, B2, B3, B9	Ca, K, Fe, Mg	10–15g

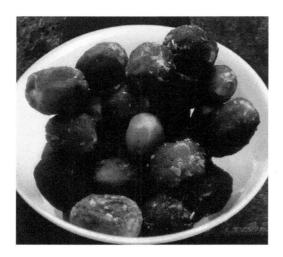

Desert Date

Local Names: *Balanites; Soapberry Tree; Lalob; Heglig; Aduwa; Kielege; Dattier du Desert; Zegene; Ader; Ghossa; Mjunju; Corona de Jesus;*

Botanical Information: *Balanites aegyptiaca (Zygophyllaceae)*

Desert date is one of the oldest recorded fruit-bearing trees, and despite its status as a 'lost crop', this tree has been around for more than 4,000 years. The trees take more than five years to bear fruit, but they can live for up to 100 years, providing many years of productivity.

Desert date is native to the arid lands of the Sahel, but its distribution ranges from Senegal and Mauritania, through Sudan, Ethiopia and Somalia, and as far south as South Africa. Desert date also grows in other arid and semi-arid parts of the world, including the Arabian Peninsula, Israel, Jordan, Iran, Pakistan and the Thar Desert in India. It was also introduced into a number of Caribbean islands including Puerto Rico and Curacao, where some trees still survive.

This small tree is drought-resistant, with a long taproot that can provide for the tree's needs once it locates underground water. It begins to branch low on the trunk, long thorns (5–8 cms) occur on the branches, and the yellowish-green flowers appear where the leaflets meet the branches. The grey-brown bark of the tree has many vertical fissures, which exude a gum when cut deeply, and helps to protect the tree from the fires that break out from time to time on the dry savannah.

Although its English name is 'desert date', this fruit is not related to the better-known date. This date is a small, plum-like drupe, which is green and becomes yellow to brown when ripe. The thin, fibrous flesh covers a light-brown, oval seed about 2 cms long. The desert date is well used wherever it grows but is generally under-utilised, given the many benefits the tree offers, not just to people and animals but also to the environment.

The desert date tree was chosen as one of the main trees to be planted in Senegal as part of the Great Green Wall (GGW) project. Due to its history across the Sahel, it would be surprising if other countries involved in that initiative have not included this resilient and bountiful tree in the fight to halt the progress of desertification.

Food Products

Desert date is eaten mostly fresh or sun-dried for later use in areas where little else is available. The taste of the fruit can vary from bittersweet to bitter and is relished by children and adults alike. The flesh of the fruit contains high levels of protein, especially for a fruit, and is comparable to levels found in some grains. There are variations in the amount of protein, dependent on soil and other conditions, but even at the lower estimates, desert date is a useful and much-needed source of protein.

Most of the carbohydrates in desert date comes from sugars, which become more concentrated as the fruit dries. This unassuming fruit has vitamins C and B and many essential and trace minerals, as well as a high fibre content. The fruit is added to cooked dishes as well as to beverages, some of which are fermented to make drinks with alcoholic content.

The most nutritious part of the desert date is the seed kernel, which, after hulling (not easy) and other processes, can be used in a variety of ways. The seed kernel needs to be boiled to reduce the bitter principle and improve the taste; they can then be roasted or ground and added to soups.

A tasty spread similar in taste to peanut butter can also be made from the roasted seeds, which are rich in protein, vitamins and minerals. With appropriate basic technology, it could be possible to get a concentrate from the dried fruit, and due to its high protein content, a concentrate could also be made from the seed kernel.

Another product of the seed kernel is a rich, golden-yellow oil that compares favourably to peanut or soya bean oil and is high in

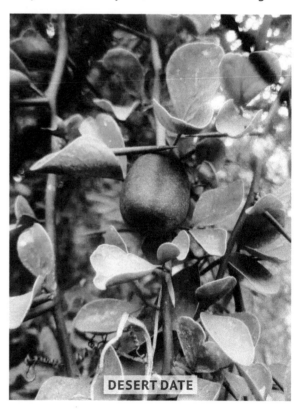

DESERT DATE

unsaturated fats. Even more important is the fact that in many areas where desert date grows, it is likely to be the only or one of few sources of dietary fat. With the exception of shea, which will be featured later, across most of the arid savannah, there are not many plants that produce oil that meets the criteria for cooking oils such as smell, taste (or lack of it, which can be a good thing for oil) and having a high smoking point.

The flowers of the tree are also cooked in some communities, as are the young leaves, which are boiled first before being fried or added to stews. Even the gum exuded from the bark is used like chewing gum, having a fairly sweet flavour.

Medicinal Properties

As can be seen from the nutritional profile of the desert date tree and its products, it can contribute to overall health improvement. Extracts from either the fruit or the seed could be made into functional food products with a range of applications, including for people living with diabetes and other cardiovascular illnesses or for those who just want to eat healthily.

All parts of the desert date are said to have medicinal properties and are used widely as such. An extract of the leaves has antibacterial properties, and the resin or gum from the bark is mixed with other herbs to treat chest pains.

The saponins, in particular diosgenin, which are present in the seed meal left after oil extraction, are precursors for steroids used in the commercial production of cortisone, contraceptive pills, oestrogen and anti-inflammatory agents.

Other Uses

The seed oil has long been used for skin and hair care, and recent research has reported that it is not only moisturising but also has antifungal and antimicrobial properties.

There are high levels of saponins in all parts of the fruits, and there is a long tradition of making soap from parts of the plant and fruit and the extracted oil.

In the Sahel region, in countries like Burkina Faso, there have been initiatives to increase oil production as well as making value-added items, such as soap and skincare products. These projects have contributed to the income of those involved, mainly women, and point to the potential that the desert date has.

Apart from direct use of the extracts of various parts of the tree for medicinal purposes, bark and fruit extracts help to kill the snails which host the worms that cause snail fever or bilharzia. The extract also kills the fleas which harbour the guinea worm eggs that cause a painful chronic illness.

The main use outside of human consumption is as animal fodder, especially in areas that often have little but acacia trees. Animals eat the leaves and fallen fruits, which provide them with a range of key nutrients.

The wood of the tree is used for carving small items but is valued as a fuel because it burns with little smoke and makes excellent high-energy charcoal, plus the seed shells are also used as a fuel.

It is evident that the desert date has huge potential, mostly unfulfilled, to improve food and nutrition security, environmental protection and soil regeneration, reduce desertification and produce a range of products that can help to develop the people and communities in the areas where the tree grows. These areas face numerous social and economic challenges, and the humble desert date has a role to play in strategies to address them.

History/Lore

Desert date is an ancient food crop that has not had any profile outside its region of usage. Both the fruits and the seed oil were highly prized in Ancient Egypt, and there are records of these from more than 4,000 years ago. In fact, samples of dried-out fruits were found in a pharaoh's tomb dating from the 12th Dynasty.

Given all we now know about this tree, its fruits, seeds, oil and other products, it is not that strange that it would have been highly sought after even in ancient times. The oil, usually marketed as *Balanites* (its botanical name), is still highly regarded across Africa and the Middle East for its many health and cosmetic properties.

The importance of desert date to the communities in which it grows cannot be overstated, and it has been like this for thousands of years – even more so now as desertification and climate change affect crops. This is exemplified by a proverb from the old Bornu empire that says 'A bito tree [desert date] and a milk cow are worth the same'.

Nutrition Information

Part of Plant	Protein	Carbohydrates	Fats	Vitamins	Minerals	Fibre
Fruit Pulp	7–10g	35–50g	1g>	C, B1, B2, B3, B6	Ca, Mg, Fe, K, Mn, P, Zn	5g
Leaves	8–12g	45g	2g	A, C	Ca, Mg, Fe, Zn, Mn,	12g
Flowers	15g	74g	4g	A, C	K, Ca, Mg, Zn, Fe, P	3–4g
Seeds	25–35g	8g	45g	A, E, B3, B9	Fe, P, Ca, Zn, Mg	10g

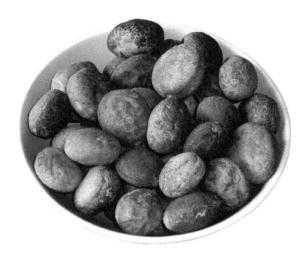

Detar

Local Names: *Sweet Detar; Dittock; Ditah; Bodo; Boto; Ofo; Tsada; Gudi; Dank; Tallow Tree, Ntamajalan; Abu Leita; Khaga, Daha; Dakpa; Tamba; Taura*

Botanical Information: *Detarium microcarpum (Fabaceae)*

There are three trees referred to as detar: *Detarium senegalense*, *Detarium microcarpum* and *Detarium macrocarpum*. While there is still some discussion regarding the botanical classification of the various detar species, these very similar trees have been classified according to their habitats and growing conditions. The information below relates to *D. microcarpum*, but it is generally accepted that much of this should be true for the other detar types.

Detar is indigenous to Africa and occurs naturally in savannah regions of many African countries, including Benin, Senegal, Burkina Faso, Chad, Sudan, Nigeria, Cameroon, Mali and The Gambia. Detar is also found in the Caribbean, where it is called tallow tree. The trees can reach a height of over 20 metres but are more usually 5–10 metres and have a distinct greyish bark.

The dark-green leaves are compound and borne on irregular branches, which form a broad canopy that provides excellent shade in regions where daytime temperatures can exceed 35°C. Detar can tolerate periods of drought but is not drought-resistant. This valuable, multipurpose tree is usually left standing when land is cleared, sometimes

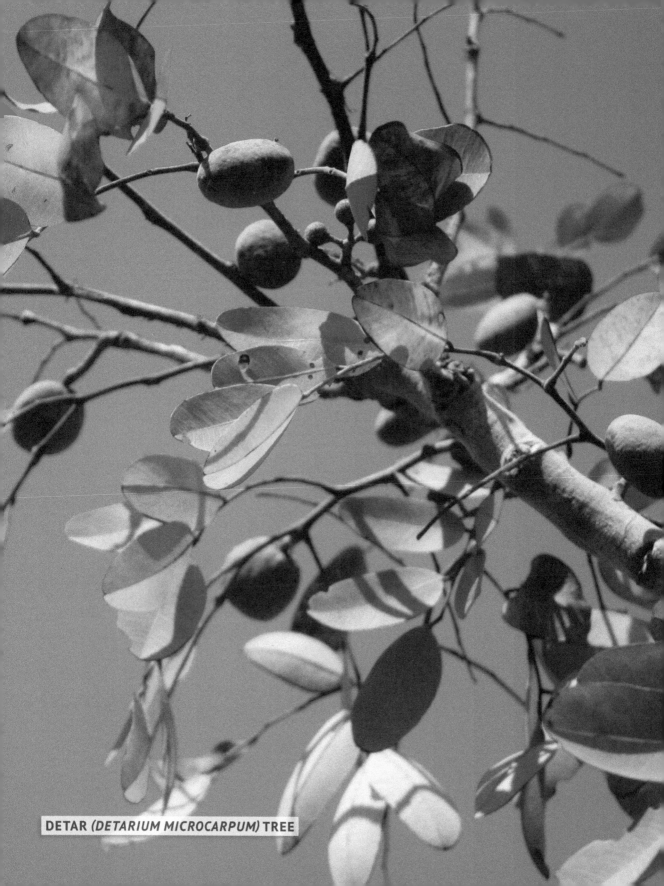

DETAR *(DETARIUM MICROCARPUM)* TREE

left standing. The tree can produce food, oil, medicine, lumber, fuel and other products and is valued by local communities.

The tree is related to tamarind and produces huge quantities (up to 7 kg per tree) of a round fruit (4x2.5 cms), which has a crisp shell that gets harder as it dries – a quality that contributes to a longer shelf life. Inside the shell is a single seed covered in a green, flaky/powdery pulp that has a sweet, tangy flavour. The seed has a sweet fragrance and has many uses.

Food Products

Detar is eaten fresh where it grows and in neighbouring areas and is also dried and sold in markets and street side stalls further from their native habitats. When the fruits are properly dried and stored in jute bags, they can be kept for up to three years. Detar has a low moisture content (estimated at 11%), which is an indicator of safe storage without deterioration.

The fruit pulp is used in various porridges and beverages as a sugar substitute, and in parts of West Africa, there are bottled juice drinks made from detar. It is also possible to find jams, purées and concentrates made from detar. It can be boiled – alone or combined with other fruits – and strained and dried to make a kind of fruit leather.

The vitamin and mineral content of the fruit pulp can vary according to the distribution of the tree and the climatic and soil conditions where it grows. The fruit is rich in potassium, phosphorous, magnesium, iron and calcium, and has one of the highest levels of vitamin C of any known fruit.

The seed of the fruit is boiled to get to its kernel, which is then pounded or ground into a nutritious flour. This is known as ofo flour in parts of Nigeria and is added to egusi soup or cooked with green vegetables. In one study, this flour was reported to have good quality protein, and an edible oil can be extracted from the seed kernel with the residue being used for animal feed.

Medicinal Properties

Detar's high vitamin C and antioxidant levels indicate that the fruit can benefit people and communities and help to increase and improve overall health and immunity. Detar flour is now being used in combination with wheat flour to make baked goods that can help people living with diabetes. Fibre plays an important role in glycaemic control, which helps to reduce the more severe consequences of diabetes.

Freeze-dried extracts of detar pulp could be used as a natural vitamin C additive to other beverages and foodstuff, which could benefit from biofortification. Detar has a higher vitamin C content than acerola cherries, which are currently one of the main sources of this vitamin in the food and beverage industry.

The bark, leaves, roots and fruits of detar are used in traditional medicine in the areas where the tree grows for a wide array of illnesses and health conditions. Extracts of the leaves, twigs and roots are used topically for wounds and skin problems, as these parts of the tree are reputed to have antimicrobial properties.

Other Uses

The wood of the detar tree is highly sought after and is sometimes called African Mahogany, due to the colour of its heartwood, although there are a number of trees with this same 'title'. The wood is used in housebuilding, furniture making and carving as well as for fuel as firewood and charcoal.

The seeds, which have a pleasant fragrance, are used to make necklaces and sometimes burnt as incense. The gum that exudes from the bark also has a pleasant smell when burnt and is used to refresh clothes and to repel insects, especially mosquitoes. Detar leaves are used for roofing material and in mask making as well as to make a good quality fertiliser.

History/Lore

Among the Igbo people of Nigeria, the detar tree is called 'Ofo' and has a very privileged role in their culture. It is regarded as a 'holy tree', which is said to have grown in God's compound. It is not only widely used for food and medicine but is also central to important spiritual and ritual events and practices.

Anyone who holds the Ofo staff has to exhibit qualities of truthfulness and impartiality in daily life as well as in important situations; it is a symbol of justice. Even in daily rituals such as prayers, the head of the household traditionally leads these and uses the Ofo staff throughout to punctuate and emphasise key points of the prayers.

Nutrition Information

Part of Plant	Protein	Carbohydrates	Fats	Vitamins	Minerals	Fibre
Fruit Pulp	4–6g	65g	2g	C, E, B2, B9	Ca, Fe, K, Mg, Zn, P, Mn	10–15g
Seed Flour	12–15g	35g	10–15g	A, C, D, B1, B3, B6	Fe, Mg, Ca, K, P	3g

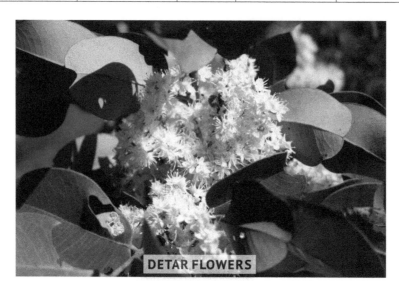

DETAR FLOWERS

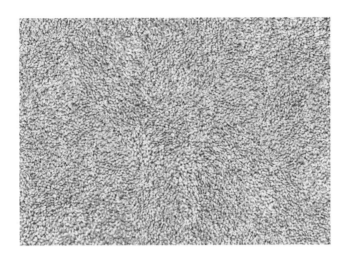

Fonio

Local Names: *Acha; Fundi; Hungry Rice; Findi; Sereme; Fini; Findo; Kpendo; Podgi; Pom; Eboniaye; Afio-warun*

Botanical Information: *Digitaria excilis; Digitaria iburua (Gramaceae)*

Fonio is an annual cereal crop that is indigenous to West Africa, said to be the oldest African cereal. It is grown for both its grain and the usefulness of the straw itself. Across the savannah regions where it is cultivated, fonio is still an important staple or major food crop for the local populations. The grain is cultivated from Cape Verde, off the coast of West Africa in a broad swathe across the Sahel and down to Lake Chad.

There are two distinct types, with the *D. iburua* being a more recent discovery from a region of Northern Nigeria. Although distinguished by colour, with *D. excilis* referred to as white fonio and *D. iburua* as black fonio, variations in the colour of the grain occur in both types. They reach a height of 40–120 cms, and the grains bear on a panicle that sometimes resembles lacy fingers.

The plant is particularly well regarded for the short time it takes to mature, which, dependent on conditions and variety, can be ready to harvest within 10 weeks, but most take 3–4 months. The plant often grows on poor, sandy and stony soils and is able to thrive with little or no rain. Fonio grows in lowlands and upland in places such as Plateau State in Nigeria and the Fouta Djallon Plateau in Guinea. In the Dominican Republic in the Caribbean, fonio grows in different soils and climatic conditions

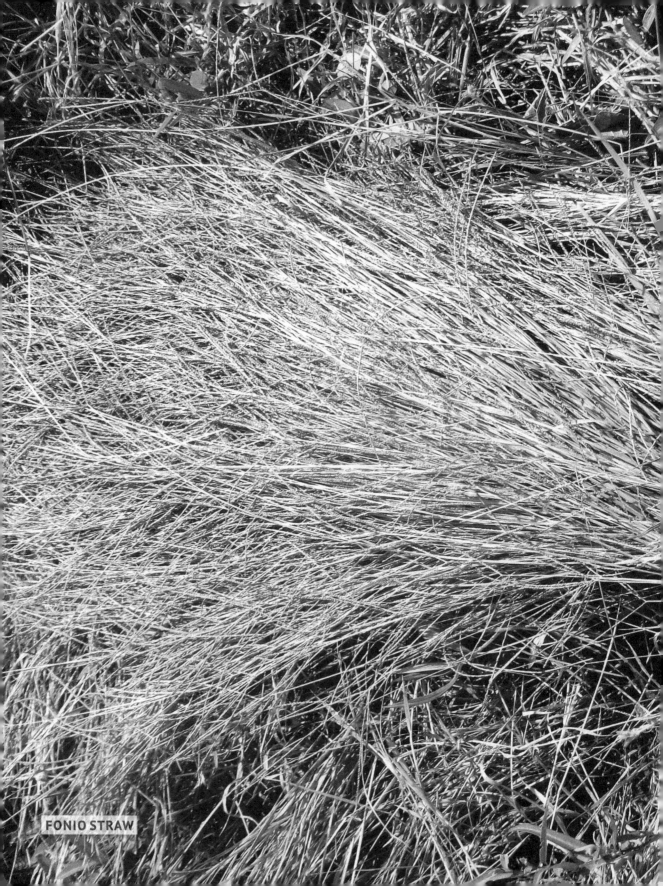

FONIO STRAW

and is valued for its ability to mature quickly and survive seasonal droughts.

Food Products

Fonio as a whole grain is comparable to rice, maize, millet or sorghum but has more essential amino acids in its protein. Fonio is rich in carbohydrates, high in fibre and is a good source of vitamins B1 and 3 and minerals such as iron, calcium, and magnesium and potassium among others.

Fonio is prepared as a whole grain like rice or couscous and despite being referred to as 'hungry rice' by some, it is given pride of place in rituals and special occasions. The taste is mild, nutty and takes on the flavour of spices very well. It is either eaten as a meal by itself when cooked with vegetables or as an accompaniment to meat or fish dishes. Fonio can also be ground into flour and used either alone or in combination with other cereals or legumes to make various baked, boiled or fermented products.

Fonio is used in the Dominican Republic in similar ways to West Africa, as a cereal or flour and made into a variety of goods or fermented to make beverages. Fonio is seen as more of a gourmet food than rice and is highly valued as an aphrodisiac, with demand consistently outstripping supply. Farmers therefore get higher prices for this grain than for others they grow.

In December 2018, the European Union officially approved fonio as an innovative and healthy ingredient, giving a modern seal of approval to an ancient grain.

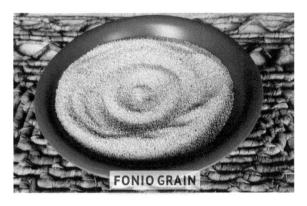

FONIO GRAIN

Medicinal Properties

Due to the properties of the starches in fonio, it is being incorporated into nutraceutical or functional food products that can help to control blood sugar levels for people living with diabetes. Its high fibre profile can also contribute to improved cardiovascular and colon health.

Other Uses

The husk of the grain and the stalks and grass are used for animal food. In fact, fonio is grown in the Americas and other places for animal feed and not for human consumption!

The stalks and grass are also used for fuel, often in places where there are few sources of firewood or other fuel.

History/Lore

Fonio grains have been found in the tomb of an Egyptian Pharaoh, and it has traditionally been regarded as the food of royals in the Sahel region going back thousands of years. The Dogon people of Mali have evolved their own unique cosmology, in which the fonio grain is of great significance. According to their beliefs, the entire universe emerged from a fonio seed, which they regard as the basic atom of creation. It still plays a very important role in their religious and cultural ceremonies.

Fonio was one of a number of crops that were brought from West Africa to the New World during the centuries of the transatlantic trade in enslaved Africans. It was cultivated in many territories in South America and the Caribbean, usually as subsistence food for the enslaved people. It was recorded and illustrated as one of the African food crops that were present in Suriname in 1590 and was an important food source for Maroon communities in the interior of Suriname. However, rice, including the original rice brought from West Africa, increased in importance and dominated food production, so little fonio is grown there now.

This ancient grain is recorded as having been in the Dominican Republic since the 16th century. Fonio is known as *funde* there, which is similar to the grain's name and its variants in West Africa. Although it was left mostly to grow wild, fonio has always featured in particular cultural and religious ceremonies and events among the African-Dominicans.

Many of the dishes consumed at these events have changed little over the centuries and are similar to traditional West African ways of preparation. The plant has been rediscovered and has gained in popularity as a profitable crop for the farmers who grow it and is highly prized for its many properties, including its taste and nutritive value. In the 1940s and 50s, the then President Rafael Trujillo and other high-profile personalities were big advocates of the grain's ability to improve virility. *Funde* is still regarded as an aphrodisiac in the Dominican Republic.

Nutrition Information

Part of Plant	Protein	Carbohydrates	Fats	Vitamins	Minerals	Fibre
Grain	7–10g	75g	2g>	B1, B2, B3	Fe, Ca, P, Mg, Mn, Zn	5g

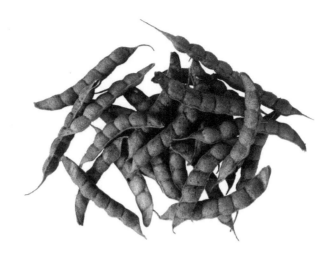

Gungo Peas

Local Names: *Pigeon Peas; Congo Peas; Arhar; Pois d'Angole; Tur Dhal; Red Gram; Gandule; Tree Bean; No Eye Pea; Kardis; Pwa Kongo*

Botanical Information: *Cajanus cajan (Fabaceae)*

Gungo is a multipurpose leguminous shrub, whose origin is said to be in South Asia; it eventually appeared in Central and West Africa more than four thousand years ago. During the transatlantic trade in enslaved Africans, gungo made its way to the Caribbean and Americas. The plant is now grown in many semi-arid, sub-tropical and tropical parts of the world. India is the largest producer, but Kenya, Malawi, Mozambique and a number of countries in the Caribbean and Americas also produce significant amounts annually.

The shrub or small tree can reach up to 5 metres high, but most trees are 2–3 metres,

with bright-yellow flowers, which are sometimes streaked or blotched with red or purple. These variations occur in the flat pods, which range from green to purple and can contain anywhere from 2–9 peas; these too come in a variety of colours and patterns.

Gungo is one of the most drought-tolerant legumes, mainly due to its roots, which go deep to both attract water as well as bringing minerals from lower down in the soil to the surface. The plant has high nitrogen-fixing ability so is good for intercropping, as it will improve the quality of the soil where it grows.

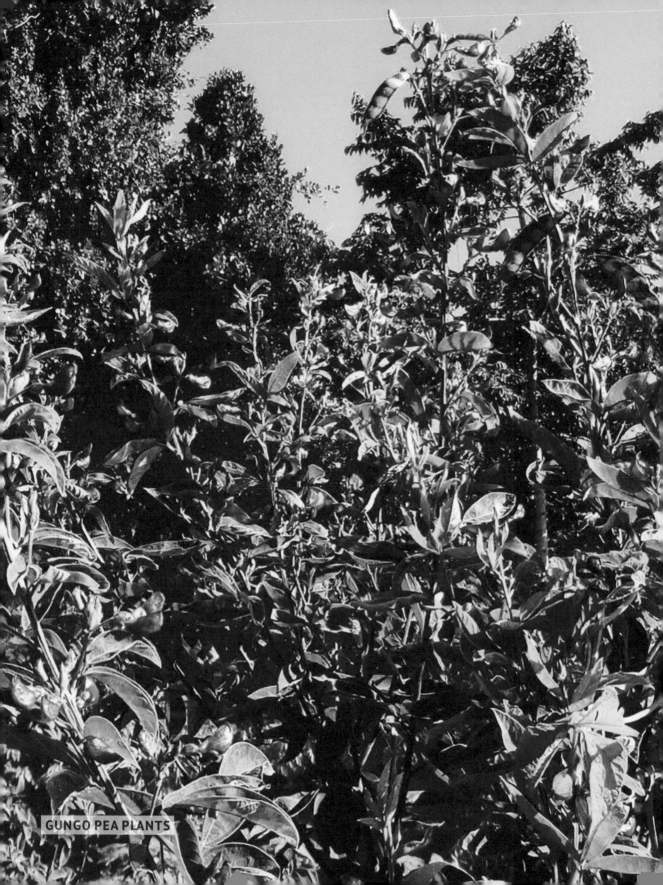

GUNGO PEA PLANTS

Food Products

Gungo peas can be eaten at different stages of growth and in many different ways, depending on custom and preference. In many countries where it is cultivated, the fresh peas are cooked like a vegetable and eaten either by themselves or as part of other recipes. The immature pod is used like French beans in curries and stews, but the mature dried peas are the most widely used. In India, the dried peas are stripped of the seedcoat and cooked as dhal or ground into a flour, which is used in combination with other flours to make baked and other goods, including snacks, noodles and functional foods.

Gungo is rich in protein, fibre, B vitamins and minerals such as iron, phosphorous, magnesium and potassium. In parts of India and neighbouring countries, dhal and flour from gungo peas are key staples. In the Caribbean and Central and South America, the fresh or dried peas are cooked with rice and served on Sundays or special occasions. Due to modern processing methods, immature gungo peas can be frozen or canned, making them accessible to diasporan communities and others far from where the peas grow.

Medicinal Properties

All parts of the gungo tree are used in herbal medicine in India, China, Africa and the Americas. Traditionally, the leaves are used internally and externally as an anti-inflammatory, for pain relief and as a broad-spectrum antimicrobial. Modern research into the properties and actions of extracts of the leaves, roots and seeds of the gungo tree has led to promising developments into potential therapeutic products for sickle cell disorders.

One such product is Ciklavit, which was developed by two Nigerian professors from gungo peas and is said to contribute to relieving symptoms of sickling. There has also been development of both therapeutic and nutraceutical products to manage diabetes and other cardiovascular conditions. Research into the medicinal potential of the plant continues in different parts of the world, and more health-giving products are likely to result.

Other Uses

The gungo tree as stated earlier is beneficial to soil not just for nitrogen fixing but also for providing green manure and shade for smaller plants, again useful when intercropping. The tree is planted as a windbreak, where necessary, and as living fences. The trees are also planted just to provide forage for animals. All parts of the gungo tree are useful for animal nutrition, either as is or in combination with other plants and grains.

Historically, the peas have been used to feed birds, including domestic fowl, hence one of the names for the plant – pigeon peas. There are continued initiatives to further develop the role of gungo peas in human and animal food and nutrition as well as in environmental protection and improvement.

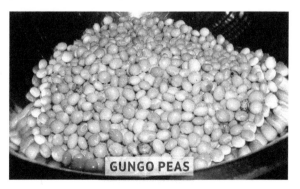
GUNGO PEAS

History/Lore

It has been well documented that many African cultural and other practices have come down through time or have been adapted to suit new situations. This is true for practices involving gungo peas' role in burial and post-burial rites. The main aim of these was to ensure that the dead person remains in the place of the dead, and these rites seem to occur both in parts of Africa and in the Caribbean.

Just as particular herbs are planted strategically in spaces where people live, with the main purpose of preventing the entry of spirits, gungo was planted near burial sites to encourage the dead to follow the path of the roots of the shrub – downwards.

In rural Jamaica, it was common practice, shortly after the burial, to tie three gungo peas in a new piece of calico, which would then be taken to the site of the grave shortly before the time of day that the person had died. They would then dig a hole and bury the tied-up peas and say the following: "Yu tan deh wid dis," which means "You must stay where this is buried."

Nutrition Information

Part of Plant	Protein	Carbohydrates	Fats	Vitamins	Minerals	Fibre
Fresh Peas	11g	45g	2g>	A, C, K, B1, B2, B3, B6, B9	Fe, P, Mg, K, Zn, Ca	8–10g
Dried Peas	20–25g	55g	3g>	A, C, K, E, B1, B2, B3, B5, B6, B9	Ca, Fe, Mg, K, P, Se, Mn	10–15g
Dhal	20g	60g	2g>	A, B1, B2, B3	Ca, Fe, Mg, Zn, K	2g
Seed Flour	18–25g	60g	2g>	A, B1, B2, B3	Fe, Ca, P, Mg, Zn	4g

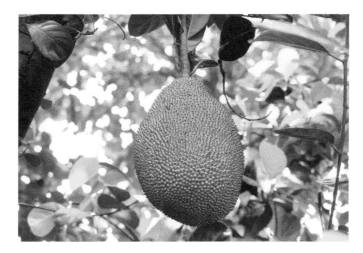

Jackfruit

Local Names: *Jak; Ceylon Jack; Katahal; Nangka; Fenesi; Kanoon; Mit; Phanas*

Botanical Information: *Artocarpus heterophyllus (Moraceae)*

Jackfruit is a stately, attractive, evergreen tree with a dense crown. The fast-growing tree can reach a height of 25 metres but is usually 5 – 15 metres high, with dark-green, glossy leaves that are thick and rubbery. Jackfruit is native to South and Southeast Asia, and countries in that area are still the major growers, but the tree now grows in East Africa, The Caribbean, Central and South America, Australia and parts of the Pacific region.

The tree can grow in a variety of soil types but needs regular rainfall throughout its life cycle. Jackfruit can survive short, seasonal drought, and mature trees are hardier than the young ones, but the tree does not thrive in areas with less than 1,500 mm annual rainfall.

Jackfruit begins to flower after two years and can fruit within three years but might take as long as five years. Although the flowers bear in abundance, a smaller proportion develop into fruits. These usually occur on the branches of the tree in younger specimens; on older trees, fruits bear on the trunk and even on the roots. In fact, there have been rare cases where the fruit has actually occurred on the roots underground. All parts of the tree, including the fruit, contain a sticky, white latex.

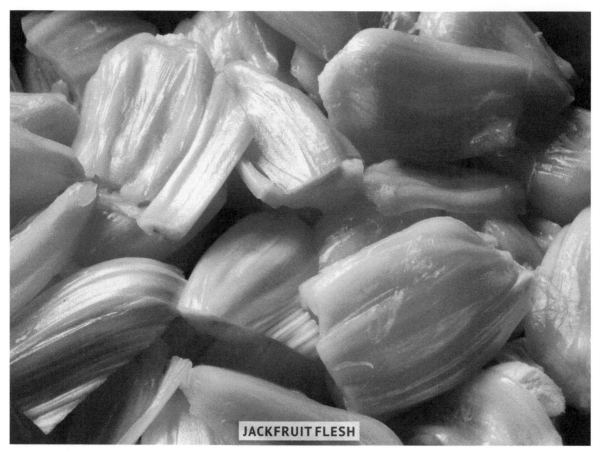

JACKFRUIT FLESH

Jackfruit is the largest tree-borne fruit in the world, measuring up to 1 metre long and weighing up to 50 kg, although most fruits are 4–10 kg. The tree is related to the breadfruit and has a similar outer rind, with a distinctive surface that is somewhere between bumpy and spiky. Inside, there is a thick inner, fibrous flesh enclosing numerous bulbs that contain a single seed in each. The smooth seed is itself covered by a thin, pale-brown membrane.

Another key feature is the number of fruits that a tree can bear, with some producing 100–200 per year. There are many varieties of jackfruit, some having been bred for particular properties, such as yield, taste, texture and, increasingly, potential for processing for added value.

One of the defining features of the jackfruit is its very distinctive odour when ripe. It is a smell that some people find unpleasant and which others like. Once the mature fruit is cut open, the odour tends to dissipate, and the dried fruit bulbs have little or no smell at all.

Food Products

As mentioned earlier, jackfruits are – even at their smallest – large fruits, but not all of the fruit is readily edible, at least not raw. The fruit does, however, offer a range of food options that make it a great candidate for food and nutrition security. Jackfruit is made up of more than 50% of a thick rind, the pulp accounts for 30% and the seeds about 12%, and each fruit can have tens to hundreds of seeds, again dependent on type.

The immature fruit is used in all sorts of recipes in many culinary traditions and is now becoming increasingly popular in Western, vegetarian and vegan dishes, described as a meat substitute. In some places, it is referred to as 'tree mutton'. At most stages of maturity, there is a lot of latex in jackfruit, which needs to be handled with care because it is so sticky. Best advice: use lots of oil on hands and knives.

Jackfruit is mostly eaten when the fruit is ripe, either fresh from the tree or made into any number of delicious beverages, desserts and confectioneries. The fruit is rich in vitamins A, C and B1 and 2, with high levels of calcium, iron, zinc and phosphorous, with a little protein, less than the immature fruit. The dried fruit makes a tasty snack, as an alternative to dried mango and pineapple.

The seeds are widely eaten roasted, boiled, mashed and fried or added to stews, curries and other dishes. They have useful amounts of protein, fat and carbohydrates and a number of B vitamins. Jackfruit seed can also be dried, ground and made into a flour that can be used in combination with other cereals or seed flours to make baked and other functional products. The seed flour contains protein, B vitamins and minerals including calcium, iron and potassium.

Jackfruit provides many nutrients from its various parts and at different stages of maturity, with little additional inputs and minimal care. This tree should be planted wherever it is able to grow, primarily for its contribution to nutrition, but there will also be added benefits, given its many uses.

Medicinal Properties

The high vitamin contents in the different parts of the jackfruit will contribute to overall health improvement, and in many areas where there are high rates of VAD, this fruit could be especially effective. The high levels of antioxidants can also help to prevent a range of inflammatory and other chronic conditions.

In all cultures where jackfruit grows, parts of the tree and fruits are used to treat a variety of illnesses and health conditions. The bark of the roots and leaves are used to treat wounds and skin problems. The seeds are also said to have aphrodisiac properties.

Other Uses

Latex from the tree parts has a variety of applications and uses, including varnishes, as it is high in resins. It is also used generally as an adhesive for china or earthenware and to caulk metal and other utensils such as buckets, pots and pans.

The tree is planted in many countries primarily for its wood, which is well regarded for carving, furniture and construction. An extract from the heartwood is used to produce a rich, yellow dye, the small branches and twigs are used for firewood and old roots are highly sought after by artisans.

Jackfruit is a good candidate for reforestation, as it serves many purposes and helps to reduce soil erosion and also control flooding. It works well being intercropped with either fast-growing fruit trees or cash crops and can provide valuable shade for crops, people and animals.

History/Lore

Jackfruit has a long history in South and Southeast Asia, where the fruit ranks only behind banana and mango in popularity. Its wood has traditionally been used to make carvings of revered gods and goddesses and special musical instruments.

Towards the end of the 18th century, the New World was still a battleground for the European countries fighting to control their newly 'discovered' territories. Britain at the time seemed to rule the waves, controlling 13 colonies in America and parts of Canada, as well as a number of Caribbean islands.

The French and Spanish were their main rivals, and by 1781, they began their grand scheme to invade and capture Jamaica, which was at that time the prize of the British colonies. The revenue coming from the island was more than that of the 13 colonies of America.

They fought the decisive Battle of the Saintes in 1782, which the British naval forces won. In that same year, a French ship carrying jackfruit plants to Martinique was captured by the British Navy and taken to Jamaica. These were the first known trees to be grown in the Caribbean, and today, jackfruit trees can be found across Jamaica and other Caribbean islands, including Martinique.

Nutrition Information

Part of Plant	Protein	Carbohydrates	Fats	Vitamins	Minerals	Fibre
Immature Fruit	2–3g	10g	1g>	A, C, B1, B2, B3, B5, B6, B9	Ca, K, Fe, P	3–5g
Ripe Fruit Pulp	1–2g	20g	1g>	A, C, B1, B2, B3, B5, B6, B9	Ca, Mg, Fe, P,	2g
Seed	5g	25–35g	1g>	A, B1, B2, B3, B5, B6, B9	Ca, Mg, Fe, K, P, Mn, Zn	3g
Seed Flour	9g	70g	1g	A, B1, B2, B3, B5, B6, B9	Ca, P, K, Fe, Mg, Mn, Zn	3g

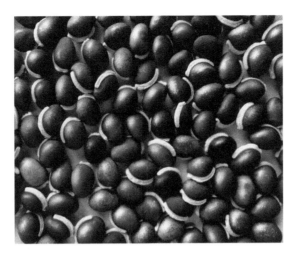

Lablab

Local Names: *Hyacinth Bean; Bonavista Bean; Chicharos; Seem; Njahe; Agaya; Kerana; Fiwi; Amora-guaya; Jefferson Bean*

Botanical Information: *Lablab purpureus (Fabaceae)*

Lablab is a multipurpose legume crop that has a long history as food, fodder and more across many continents for thousands of years. The plant can be erect, trailing or climbing, and can range from 2–6 metres in length. It is thought, based on the occurrence of wild ancestors of the species, that lablab originated in Africa in the eastern Sahel, eventually spreading to South and Southeast Asia and beyond. There are said to be more than a hundred varieties, based on differences in shape, size and colour of pods, seeds, flowers, leaves and other characteristics.

Lablab is widely distributed across many tropical, subtropical and even temperate parts of the world, including South and Central America, and can tolerate a wide variety of soil types, even toxic aluminium soils. Experts suggest that the plant has adapted to the varied environmental and climatic conditions in which it finds itself, and this has given rise to the wide variation in the characteristics of lablab. This legume grows from sea level up to 2,000 metres above sea level, in temperatures 15–40°C and with annual rainfall levels between 300–2,000 mm. It seems that the main growing condition it does not like is waterlogged soils. Lablab has very deep taproots that can extract soil water from 2 metres depth and is said to be able to cope better with drought than even cow peas (*Vigna unguiculata*).

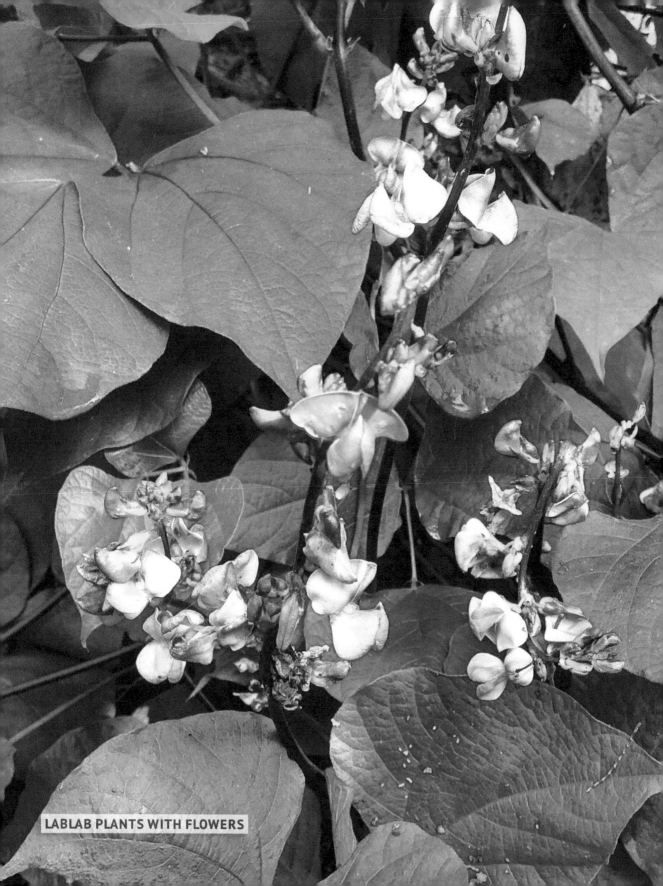

LABLAB PLANTS WITH FLOWERS

The leaves occur in threes (trifoliate), with the base of the leaves being broader than the pointed apex and are smooth on the upper surface but often hairy on the underside. Lablab leaves range in colour from pale green to purple, and the showy flowers which occur in clusters can be creamy white, pink, red or purple. The pods reflect the colour of the leaves, and the beans similarly vary in colour, as well as those that are brown, black and mottled. Most beans are ovoid in shape, and all have a distinct white helium. Although the shape and size of the pods vary, some being flatter than others, they have a curved beak at one end and contain from 2–6 beans.

Food Products

Lablab is eaten at different stages of maturity. Different parts of the plant are edible, and these can all be prepared in numerous ways, dependent on country and local preferences. Young, tender leaves are used in both East and West Africa and Southeast Asia as a vegetable and potherb.

The leaves are rich in protein, vitamins and minerals and are one of the best vegetable

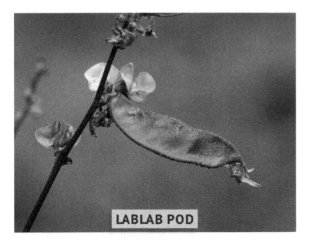

LABLAB POD

sources of iron. A few lablab varieties have been developed for primary use as a green, leafy vegetable that can be used within 40 days of sowing and which continues to produce for a few months.

The immature beans are consumed whole like string beans or mangetout so can be added to stir-fries, stews and many types of curry. They have high levels of vitamins A, K and C, minerals and fibre. Mature beans that are fresh are soaked overnight and the outer skin removed. They can be then cooked either alone or with other grains, cereals or vegetables.

Dried lablab beans are rich in many nutrients but for a variety of reasons are not currently being used as much as their benefits would suggest. In Africa and the Caribbean, the beans were used more widely in the past but has lost ground to soya beans, cow peas and other legumes. Dried lablab can also be ground into a flour, which can be used to fortify wheat or other flour to make pasta, baked goods and weaning foods.

In Indonesia, lablab is sometimes substituted for soya in making traditional, fermented tempeh. The bean can also make a curd similar to tofu, and due to the lower cost of lablab, the curd costs less.

Medicinal Properties

Nutritious food can contribute to more than just satisfying hunger and can help us to maintain good health or reduce the risks of more serious illnesses. The bean has a low sodium and high potassium content, which is helpful for high blood pressure and other cardiovascular problems.

Extracts can also be used to formulate nutraceutical products targeted at particular conditions. Wherever lablab grows, it is used in traditional herbal medicine, with the leaves being the most widely used. They are taken for various conditions, including stomach problems and to help with childbirth, and when crushed in vinegar are applied as an antidote for snake bites. Among some communities, lablab is consumed as a food to help lactating mothers.

Other Uses

Labab is mostly used outside of Africa and Asia as animal fodder or as a showy ornamental plant. In Africa, lablab is widely used as green manure and generally to improve soil conditions.

History/Lore

In the United States, lablab is often referred to as the 'Thomas Jefferson bean', and the plant is not regarded as a food crop. It is said that in 1804, Thomas Jefferson bought lablab vines from his favourite gardening supplier, Bernard McMahon. The varied colours, especially the red and purple flowers and the bean pods, are eye-catching, and the plant requires little care and few inputs for what is a great effect.

Since that time, lablab vines have been present in the vegetable garden at Jefferson's Monticello Plantation in Virginia. The fact that it was planted in the vegetable garden suggests that perhaps enslaved people on the estate were familiar with this plant from Africa and would have known how to prepare dishes with the beans or leaves. Monticello still markets lablab seeds for planting, and the plants there continue to enthral and intrigue visitors to the property.

Nutrition Information

Part of Plant	Protein	Carbohydrates	Fats	Vitamins	Minerals	Fibre
Immature Beans	3g	9g	1g>	C, A, K, B1, B2, B3, B5, B6, B9	Ca, Fe, Mg, P, Zn, K, Mn Zn	7–10g
Dried Beans	24g	60g	2g	A, B1, B2, B3, B5, B6, B9	Fe, Ca, P, Mg, Zn, K, Mn	10g
Leaves	25g		1g	A, C, D, E	Ca, Fe, K, Mg, P	12g
Bean Flour	20g	65g	1g	A, B1, B2, B3, B5, B6, B9	Fe, Ca, P, Zn	4g

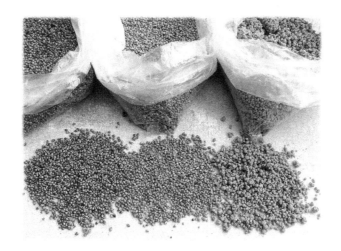

Millets

Millets are a diverse group of cereals that share some features such as their environmental adaptability and, as their name suggests, very small grains. Millets have been marginalised in terms of research and development of new varieties when compared to wheat, rice and maize.

These ancient cereals have sustained generations of people over thousands of years, often in poor and unpredictable growing conditions. Millets were mentioned in the Bible and other ancient texts as an important staple and now rank as the sixth most widely used grain after corn, rice, wheat, barley and sorghum. They continue to produce significant yields in arid and semi-arid, fertile or marginal lands, need minimum inputs and are good nutritional sources.

Given the predictions of experts about climate change, especially increases in temperatures and scarcity of water, it becomes even more urgent for crops like millet that are drought-resistant to be promoted and given a higher priority in food security policies and projects.

Two of the most important of the millets are finger millet and pearl millet, and these crops offer many benefits for people living in vulnerable areas, who often experience nutritional deficiencies. Millets and their food products could also be beneficial for the many millions in the world who are overweight, obese, or who are living with conditions such as gluten intolerance, high blood pressure, diabetes and other cardiovascular problems.

History/Lore

In ancient China, millet was one of five sacred grains, and it is thought that in those days, millet not rice was the staple of the majority of the population. Hou Ji is an honoured figure in Chinese culture and history, achieving almost god-like status. Hou Ji's name translates as

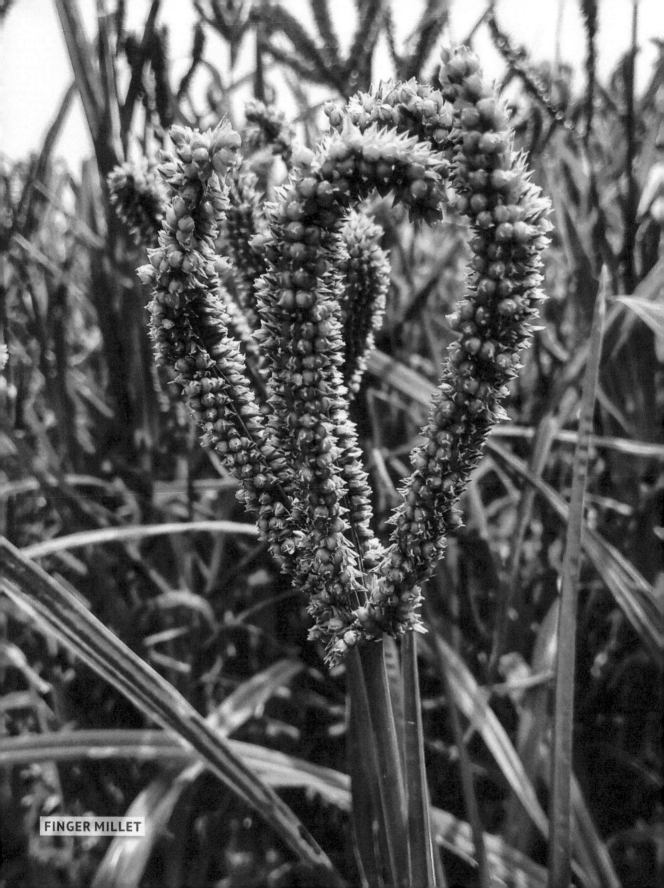
FINGER MILLET

'Lord of the Millets', and he is particularly revered for his role in the development of agriculture and the cultivation of millet.

Millets were and continue to be a favourite grain of nomadic and semi-nomadic communities, especially as some types can mature within 70 days of planting. This offers a great opportunity for the planting and harvesting of a crop, which can be stored for use when the community moves on.

Finger Millet

Local Names: *Ragi; Tamba; Telebun; Wimbi; Takuso; Petit Mil; Coracan; Tamba; Wimbi; Ulezi; Koddo; Korrakan*

Botanical Information: *Eleusine coracana (Poaceae)*

Finger millet originated in the highlands of East Africa, with the oldest grain being found near Axum in Ethiopia, dated at more than 5,000 years old. It spread from there southward as far as Mozambique and as far west as Namibia. Finger millet eventually reached India more than 2,000 years ago and is still grown in many arid and semi-arid parts of the country, with production of more than 2 million tonnes annually.

In East Africa, where it was a staple crop for centuries, finger millet has been overtaken by the introduction of maize and types of wheat, which require many costly inputs. There is still, however, significant cultivation of the cereal in Kenya, Zimbabwe and Uganda. Even in West Africa, where finger millet was not widely grown, there has been an increase in production in parts of Senegal, Niger and Nigeria. Finger millet can adapt to varying climatic and soil conditions and thrives where other cereals fail, which should encourage wider cultivation of this ancient grain.

Finger millet is an annual plant with narrow, grass-like leaves and has a lot of tillers, which produce multiple seed heads. These heads consist of spikes that look like fingers in a fist, hence the common English name. The tiny grains bear on these spikes, giving the plant its distinctive look. Finger Millet can, depending on variety, be from 0.5–1.5 metres high and also varies in the time it takes from planting to maturity, from 90–120 days. There are white, red and brown coloured grains, and preference is based on what the grain is being used for, rather than differences in nutritional value.

The very small size of the grain offers advantages and disadvantages during harvest and post-harvest in terms of storage and processing. The grain can be stored for 5–10 years, due to its resistance to insects, but can be problematic to mill and process.

Food Products

Finger millet is sometimes regarded in both India and in parts of Africa as 'famine food' and is one of the reasons why it has not been as well promoted as it should be, given its many attributes. Despite the fact that millions of people rely on finger millet as their staple food, there are many more who could be benefitting from regular consumption of the various foods that can be made from this cereal.

Protein content in finger millet varies according to type and growing conditions, but it has a well-balanced amino acid profile. It has the highest calcium content of all cereals and also has good amounts of iron, magnesium, manganese and phosphorous.

The grains are dried, fermented or malted and can be cooked whole or cracked and used like rice or couscous and eaten with stews and sauces. Finger millet can also be milled/ground into flour: in India, this is used to make chapatis (unleavened flatbreads); in parts of East Africa, the flour is made into a stiff porridge like pap or ugali (maize).

Apart from the nutritional punch that finger millet packs, it also has a pleasant, nutty taste and can be made into many products either alone or in combination with other grains or starches. Breads, buns, biscuits, breakfast cereals and cereal bars are among the products that can be made with composite flour. The flour can be from dried, fermented or malted grains.

Some types of finger millet are grown primarily for commercial production of non-alcoholic and alcoholic beverages. Finger millet is said to be second only to barley, among cereals, in its ability to hydrolyse starches, which is necessary in the fermentation process. Malting of millets and other suitable grains is being promoted by some nutrition experts as a useful method for improving the taste and flavour of these staple crops and also to increase the availability of the nutrients when consumed.

Medicinal Properties

When people have access to nutritious foods on a regular basis, their overall health improves, as does their ability to minimise or reduce the regularity and severity of disease and ill health. When foods such as finger millet are part of a varied diet, both undernourishment and malnutrition can be reduced or eliminated. As a cereal, it is gluten free so can be beneficial for people who have health conditions such as colitis and gluten sensitivity or intolerance.

The grain's high fibre content and the quality of its starches helps it to balance glucose absorption in the body, which is very useful for the management and control of diabetes. With its exceptionally high calcium content, it can be effective in treating conditions that involve calcium deficiency.

Nutrition Information

Part of Plant	Protein	Carbohydrates	Fats	Vitamins	Minerals	Fibre
Grain	7g	75g	2g>	A, E, B1, B2, B3, B9	Ca, Fe, Mg, P, Mn, Zn, K	3g
Flour	11g	75g	4.3g	B1, B2, B3	Ca, Fe, K	4g

Pearl Millet

Local Names: *Cattail Millet; Bulrush Millet; Candle Millet; Bajra; Petit Mil; Sanyo; Uwele; Gero; Mhunga; Mwere; Dukhan*

Botanical Information: *Pennisetum glaucum (Poaceae)*

Pearl millet is the staple cereal for more than 500 million people, but it has remained largely unknown outside of the regions where it is cultivated or consumed. As with finger millet, pearl millet has long been regarded as 'poor people's food' and therefore not valued. As a result, the trend in production in some places is going down.

This hardy cereal is thought to have originated more than 5,000 years ago in the savannahs of West Africa and then spread to India and other parts of South Asia. Today, Sahelian countries, such as Burkina Faso, Mali and Niger, and parts of India produce the bulk of the estimated 18 million tonnes annual global production. Pearl millet is also cultivated in Namibia, Sudan and Uganda and was a staple in parts of Southern Africa until the advent of maize.

Pearl millet is an annual grass that can be from 0.5–4 metres tall, with a profuse root system that is able to go down 3 metres into the ground. It has a slender stalk, often with tillers, and the leaves, which are similar to sugar cane, can be up to 1.5 metres long and 8 cms in width. The inflorescence also varies in size from 15 cms to 1.40 metres long and can be cylindrical in shape or can taper towards each end. The colour of the grains is usually silvery grey but can vary from white to dark brown. The length of time from planting to maturity can vary from 55–280 days, but 75–180 days is more usual.

Pearl millet is produced mainly by small-scale farmers, for whom it is a means of food security as well as a source of income when yields are good. The plant's ability to adapt to unpredictable climatic conditions and poor or marginal soil makes it a better option than maize, which requires many more inputs, especially water and fertilisers to yield significant amounts. More research needs to be done to identify and suggest solutions to problems associated with harvesting and processing pearl millet.

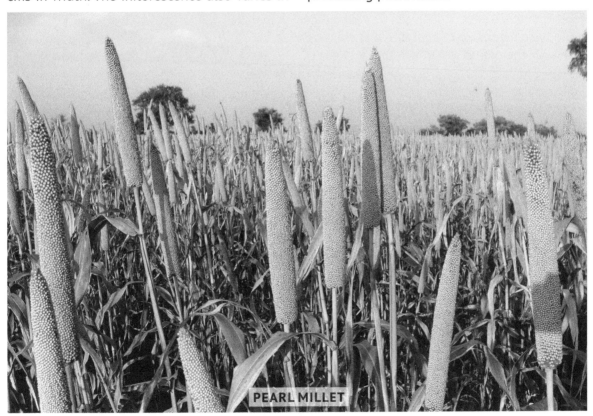
PEARL MILLET

Food Products

Pearl millet offers many nutritional benefits, as well as a wide array of possible food processing and preparation options. This cereal has a high protein content for a grain, with a well-balanced amino acid profile. It is rich in zinc, iron and potassium and is high in vitamin A. Pearl millet contains 5% fat, which is twice the amount of most cereals; this fat is 75% unsaturated and 24% saturated.

The dried grain can be cooked, whole or cracked like rice or couscous, and this can be used in savoury and sweet dishes. It can also be ground into a flour, which is used to make a stiff porridge, like toh, or to make unleavened breads like chapatis or roti in India. In Nigeria, pearl millet is fermented and used to make a dish called 'ogi' that is also used as a weaning food. Immature pearl millet can be roasted or boiled and eaten like a vegetable, and children often eat the grains straight from the stalk.

Pearl millet is becoming more widely used in brewing processes, and some strains have been developed with higher-than-average starch content. As stated in the finger millet section, malted pearl millet can be helpful in the development of foods for weaning infants and speciality nutritional products.

Other Uses

One of the main uses for pearl millet, apart from human nutrition, is for animal nutrition: parts of the plant and by-products play an important role for livestock. In many cases, pearl millet grows on some of the most marginalised lands, for example, in the Sahel region, where few cereals can survive. This adaptable crop withstands all kinds of pests, drought, sandstorms and the odd rainstorm that dumps annual rainfall in an afternoon. When the crop fails, there are no other options, and humans and livestock suffer.

Large and small ruminants eat the residue of harvested plants as well as getting damaged stalks and grains, all of which contribute to their survival when there is little else to forage. Taller stalks are used for temporary fencing, roofing and for fuel, often in places where there are few materials available for these needs. The stems are sometimes split and used in basket making.

Nutrition Information

Part of Plant	Protein	Carbohydrates	Fats	Vitamins	Minerals	Fibre
Grain	11g	70g	5g	A, B1, B2, B3, B9	Fe, Ca, Mg, Mn, P, K	2g

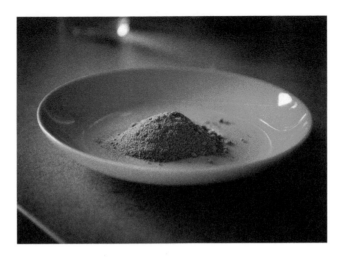

Moringa

Local Names: *Horseradish Tree; Ben Oil Tree; Drumstick Tree; Malunggay; Benzolive Tree; Senjana; Muringa*

Botanical Information: *Moringa oleifera (Moringaceae)*

Moringa is a fast-growing, perennial tree, which can reach up to 12 metres high at maturity. The tree grows best in hot, semi-arid, tropical areas and is drought-tolerant. The drooping branches have pale-green, feathery, compound leaves. The flowers range from creamy-white to yellow and bear long triangular pods, which are usually 30–50 cms in length but can exceed one metre. The pods contain between 12–35 'winged' seeds that are covered with a white membrane and have a high oil content.

Moringa has been described as 'potentially one of earth's most valuable plants'. The tree provides a veritable treasure chest of nutrients as well as other benefits. The flowers, leaves, green pods, seeds, bark and roots of the tree can be used for food, medicine and a variety of other applications.

Moringa is more widely cultivated and utilised across the Indian subcontinent, where it originated, and other parts of Asia. Although moringa has now become naturalised in most parts of Sub-Saharan Africa and the Caribbean, it is not used as widely as it should be and needs to be better incorporated in meaningful attempts at improving food security and nutrition.

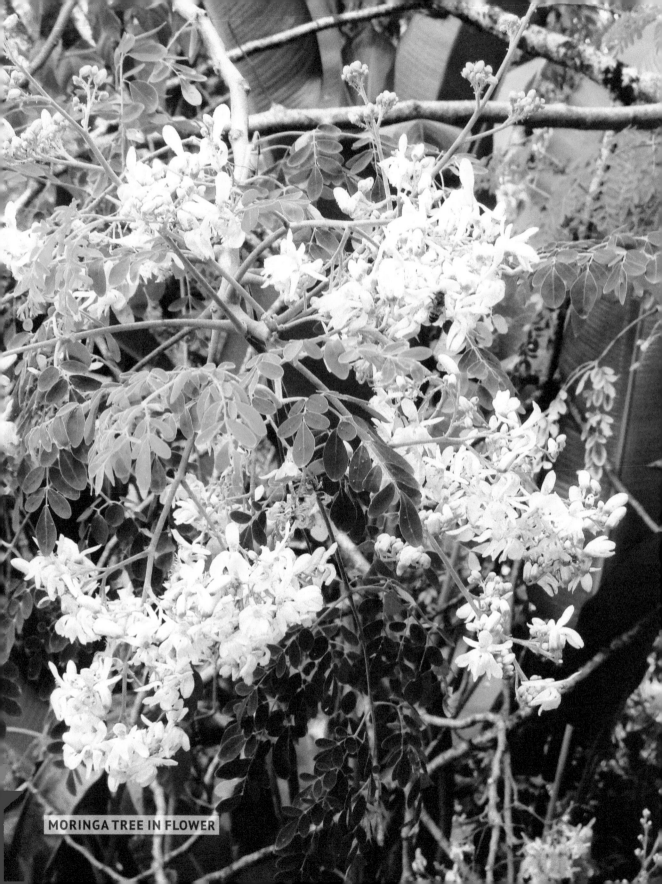

MORINGA TREE IN FLOWER

Food Products

Moringa has come to international prominence, primarily because of the wide range of both macro- and micronutrients that different parts of the tree contain. The leaves of the moringa tree can be used fresh, cooked or stored as dried powder that can last for many months without loss of nutrients. NGOs such as Trees for Life, working in developing countries, have advocated for many years to increase the use of moringa as a nutritional intervention in cases of moderate and severe malnutrition.

In terms of macronutrients, fresh raw moringa leaves contain good levels of protein and carbohydrates as well as calcium and vitamins A, B and C. The dried leaf powder contains even more protein, with a good balance of amino acids, fat and carbohydrates and has high levels of calcium, potassium, magnesium, iron and zinc. The dried leaves are particularly rich in beta-carotene as well as important plant chemicals that are beneficial for general health and disease prevention.

The young seed pod, which can be eaten like a vegetable, contains vitamin C, a range of B vitamins, amino acids and minerals, such as iron and potassium, and is higher in fibre than the fresh leaves. Moringa seeds can be eaten raw or cooked when still immature, but as they mature, they become bitter so are mostly used for oil extraction.

The seeds contain on average 40% oil, which is sweet, non-sticking, non-drying and resists rancidity. Moringa oil has a high percentage of unsaturated fats (82%) in comparison to saturated fats (13%) and is rich in essential fatty acids. The oil has a multitude of applications, but in terms of nutrition, it can be used for culinary purposes and is similar to olive oil.

Medicinal Properties

Moringa is indeed the poster tree for the interface between food and medicine. As seen above, the range of nutrients that all parts of the tree contain can contribute to improved health and nutritional status. The exceptionally high level of beta-carotene, especially in the dried leaves, could be an effective tool in reducing high rates of VAD in some populations. This could be achieved either by direct use or incorporating extracts into functional food products.

There is anecdotal and research evidence that various parts of the moringa tree have analgesic, antibacterial, antioxidant, anti-inflammatory and immuno-stimulant properties.

Other Uses

The seedcake left after oil extraction has excellent water purification properties, offering a readily available low-tech solution to a major problem in many parts of the world where scarcity of potable water occurs. Having access to adequate amounts of clean water is an important contribution to health improvement and disease prevention as well as overall economic development.

Moringa seed oil is highly prized in the cosmetic and perfume industry for its emollient qualities and its ability to absorb essential oils. It is used in the manufacture of hair and skincare products. Moringa oil, often referred to as 'ben oil' can also be used for lubrication and for lighting purposes, as it burns well and has a high smoking point.

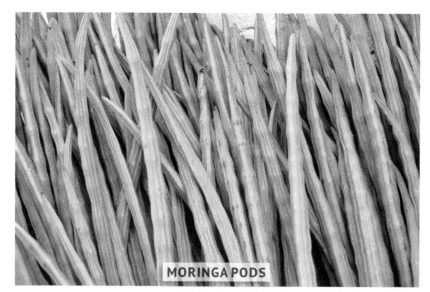
MORINGA PODS

Another important use of moringa is for animal fodder, which improves livestock production, demonstrating further just how useful this tree is. Moringa leaves, twigs and seedcake can all be sources of food for animals from cattle and sheep to chickens and rabbits.

History/Lore

Moringa was well-known in antiquity with evidence that the plant was utilised by the Ancient Egyptians, Romans and Greeks. There are records of the oil – which was called 'Baqet Oil' – being imported (from Asia) to Egypt in 3000 BC. Moringa oil was used there for medicine, cosmetic and perfumery purposes and importantly for embalming processes.

British colonialists became familiar with the tree in the Indian subcontinent, and over time, they introduced it to other parts of their empire, including Jamaica and other Caribbean islands. The British found the taste of the grated roots of the moringa plant to be similar to horseradish and in fact called it the horseradish tree. In the early 19th century, there were calls in the Jamaican Parliament for the expansion of moringa farms, which thrived on the hot southern plains of the island. These were planted mainly for the oil, which was widely used at that time in fine machinery such as watches and clocks, especially in Switzerland and Germany. Use of moringa oil declined with the growing availability of olive and palm oil.

Nutrition Information

Part of Plant	Protein	Carbohydrates	Fats	Vitamins	Minerals	Fibre
Fresh Leaves	8g	10g	2g>	A, C, E	Fe, Ca, K, P, Mg, Mn, Zn	5g
Dried Leaf Powder	23g	30–40g	7g	A, E, C, B1, B2, B3, B5, B6, B9	Fe, Ca, P, K, Mg, Zn, Mn	10g
Young Seed Pods	3g	8g	2g	A, C, B1, B2, B3, B5, B6	Ca, Fe, K, Mg, P	3g

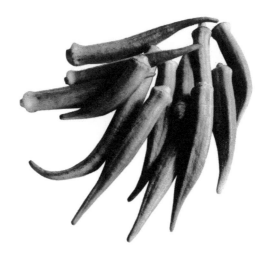

Okra

Local Names: *Gumbo; Quaibo; Bhindi; Ladies' Fingers; Bamia; Ki Ngombo; Ocro; Nkruman; Fevi; Okwuru; Kanja*

Botanical Information: *Abelmoschus esculentus (Malvaceae)*

Okra originated in North East Africa, in the region between Sudan and Ethiopia, but is now one of the most widely cultivated, tropical vegetables. It is grown in such diverse places as Southern Europe and Southeast Asia, the Caribbean and Americas and many parts of Africa. Okra is said to be one of the oldest cultivated crops, but despite being widely distributed, it is still not regarded as a popular vegetable.

There are now many varieties of okra globally, with commercial production and processing in countries like India (the leading producer), Turkey and Iran. There are still debates about how much and what types are cultivated across Africa, it is truly a pan-African crop, and reported quantities suggest that there are significant amounts of okra being grown in countries like Nigeria.

Okra is an annual, erect plant about 2 metres in height, although some varieties in Africa can be up to 5 metres tall. The main stalk of the plant, usually with a diameter of 6–10 cms, becomes woody as the plant matures. The heart-shaped, lobed leaves, which can be up to 30 cms in length, are attached to the stalk, where the flower eventually appears. The pale- to bright-yellow flowers have a red to purple base, and there are a few varieties whose flowers are shades of pink.

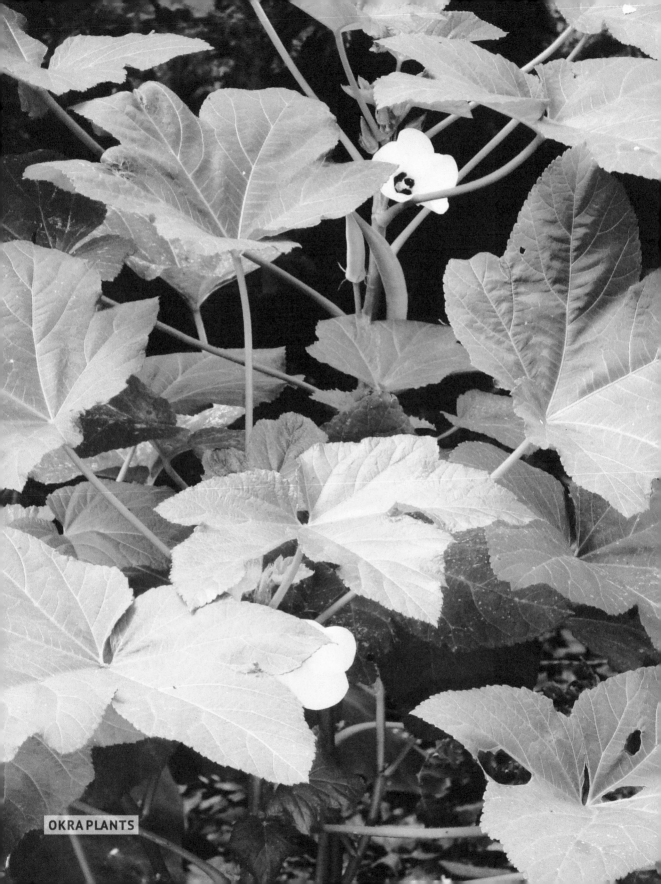

OKRA PLANTS

There are now varieties that mature more quickly than traditional types, but plants flower eight weeks after planting and quickly develop into pods or fruits, which can be picked within 5-7 days. Pods can be from 6-25 cms long and covered with fine hairs and ribs or smooth and round. The longer the pods mature, the tougher and more fibrous they become, and the seeds within, which are white when the fruit is immature, become darker and harder as they dry.

Just as the fruit grows in many diverse places, with a range of climatic conditions, it also tolerates a variety of soils. Okra is a multipurpose plant, with uses in food and other commercial production processes. With its excellent nutritional profile, it is surprising that there have not been more initiatives to increase global production.

Food Products

Okra, despite its long history and wide distribution, needs to be better promoted as a nutritional powerhouse. It grows quickly, and it is possible to pick the tender lower leaves to use as a potherb as is done in many parts of Africa and Asia. Sometimes the flowers and young fruits are added to stews and soups, but the young, tender fruits or pods are the most widely used part of the plant.

These pods are cooked in many different ways, either alone or in combination with other vegetables, pulses and grains. Okra is rich in vitamins C, K, B1 and B6 as well as minerals such as potassium, magnesium and dietary fibre. Young, fresh okras are canned and frozen on a commercial scale, and in many African countries, they are sliced and dried for later use. The mucilage or slime that is a feature of the young pods is said to be the reason that okra is not so popular; it is reduced as the pods get drier.

Okra is the key ingredient in the renowned Southern US dish called 'gumbo' and is also prepared in a variety of ways according to cultural or regional preferences. In some areas, there is a fondness to add okra to seafood dishes whereas others prefer them with meats.

For most people, that is the end of the okra story, but it is becoming more obvious that the dried okra seeds have a lot to offer. The seeds have a nutritive profile that it is similar to soya bean, with high protein and oil content. An edible oil can be extracted from the seeds, and there are a number of possible uses for the residual seedcake.

The seeds can be ground and the flour used for protein enrichment, including fortification of cereals and other goods such as a tofu-like curd and meat substitute products, currently based on soya. There have been some concerns about the presence and levels of a substance called gossypol in okra seed, but there is no clear evidence that this is a problem.

Ground, roasted okra seeds have long been enjoyed as a coffee substitute, and the absence of caffeine would benefit the health conscious.

Medicinal Properties

The main health benefits of okra are the high fibre content and the mucilage. Fibre in the diet helps to slow the absorption of blood sugar, and the mucilage also helps to improve digestion and is mildly laxative.

Mucilage is also used in many products that cater for people who suffer from chronic constipation and other digestive conditions. Currently, most of this is sourced from psyllium husks and flaxseed but could easily be extracted from okra. Okra leaves can be heated and pounded to make a poultice to help heal wounds and reduce inflammation.

Other Uses

There is a huge international market for functional products as well as for cosmetic and personal care products, of which okra's mucilage content could be a part. Currently, aloe vera is used for many topical products that require cooling, healing properties; okra could become another source on a commercial scale.

The husks and stalks of the okra plant can be used as substitute for jute and can also be used to make good quality paper and paper sizing. The high cellulose content in the okra bast fibres offers the opportunity for many commercial and industrial applications.

History/Lore

Ki ngombo is the term for okra in an Angolan language; even today in many parts of West Africa, it is called gumbo. Okra arrived in the New World soon after the first arrivals of enslaved Africans in Brazil in the 16th century and was noted in the 17th century in parts of the Caribbean. A stew of okra was referred to in the Southern states of the USA in the 1700s, particularly in South Carolina and Louisiana.

New Orleans has become the place most strongly associated with the dish called 'gumbo', which is a mix of okra, spices and seafood, and variations of it are consumed in different parts of the USA. Similar dishes are enjoyed in Senegal, Brazil and the Eastern Caribbean, where 'callaloo' is a dish made from taro leaves, okra, spices and seafood.

Nutrition Information

Part of Plant	Protein	Carbohydrates	Fats	Vitamins	Minerals	Fibre
Fruit Pod	2g	7g	1g>	A, C, K, B1, B2, B3, B6, B9	Ca, Mg, K, Fe, P,	3g
Leaves	4g	11g	1g>	A, C, B1, B2, B3	Fe, Ca, P	2g
Dried Seeds	20–25g	20–30g	20–40g	C, K, B1, B2, B3, B6, B9	K, P, Fe, Mg, Zn, Mn	10–15g
Seed Flour	23–30g	30g	15–20g	C, B1, B2, B3, B6, B9	Fe, K, P, Mg, Ca, Mn	10g

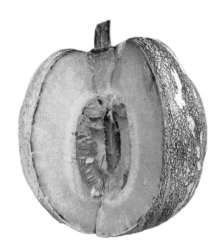

Pumpkin

Local Names: *Squash; Cushaw; Calabaza; Kadoo; Ayote; Kumra; Citrouille; Zapallos; Mboga; Pogidje; Yoogre*

Botanical Information: *Cucurbita moschata (Cucurbitaceae)*

Pumpkin is a member of a large family of plants called cucurbits, which includes melon, cucumber, chayote, gourds and various squashes. The plant is said to have originated in Central America or the northern parts of South America but has spread to tropical, sub-tropical regions and temperate parts of the world.

Pumpkin is a creeping or climbing annual vine with hairy stems and leaves that can be up to 30 cms long and 20 cms wide. These leaves often have white blotches on them and can be heart-shaped or circular. Within a few months of planting, large, bell-shaped flowers appear; these range in colour from pale yellow to orange.

The flowers soon bear fruits that can be oval, round or almost oblong and can weigh up to 40 kgs when mature. The colour of the flesh of the pumpkin ranges from pale green or yellow to deep orange, and the texture of the flesh and colour of the skin also differ according to the particular variety, climatic and soil conditions.

The centre of the pumpkin fruit is hollow with loose fibres encasing numerous seeds, depending on type, which are oval, flat and can be white to light brown, with a kernel

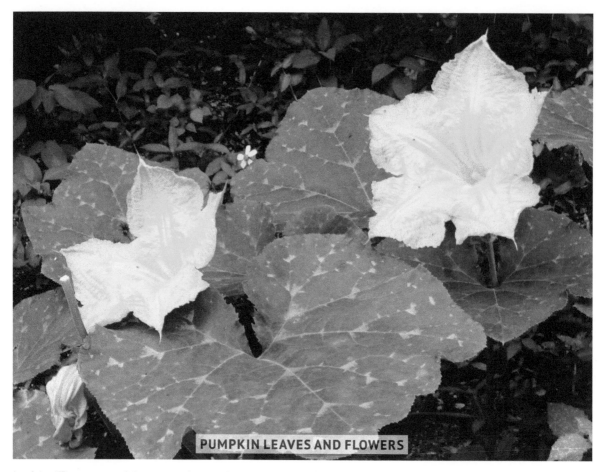

PUMPKIN LEAVES AND FLOWERS

inside. These nutritious seeds are best when the fruits are fully matured, and in some countries, they are more highly prized than the fruits themselves.

This humble vegetable can be easily grown in backyards or gardens as well as on larger tracts of land.

Food Products

This versatile vegetable has so many qualities but only seems to receive attention in popular culture once a year during Halloween, when outsize pumpkins are used for decoration and sometimes pies.

Pumpkin has a lot to offer in terms of usage, as its leaves, flowers, fruits and seeds are consumed in the many places where it grows. Pumpkin leaves are usually eaten when young and are prepared like other traditional greens. These leaves are particularly popular in Southern Africa, where they are among the main greens consumed daily. Pumpkin leaves contain protein, good quality carbohydrates and fibre as well as vitamins and minerals.

The flesh of the fruit is the most widely used part globally, usually being added to savoury soups and stews. It is also an ingredient in sweet dishes such as puddings and the famous American pumpkin pies. The flesh is rich in beta-carotene, vitamins and minerals, including calcium, potassium and magnesium. Some of these nutrients vary in amount depending on stage of maturity, soil and other conditions. For example, the carotenoids (that give the fruit its deep-orange colour) are ten times higher in mature fruits than in immature ones.

If the pumpkin has the stem intact when harvested, it can then be stored in a dry, cool place for many months, without loss of nutrients or quality. In parts of Africa and Asia, pumpkin is sliced and dried to preserve it for future use.

There have been recent initiatives to produce pumpkin flour or powder, which can be added to cereal or legume flours to make baked goods, or as a thickener in soups and stews or to smoothies to increase the nutritive value.

The seeds of the pumpkin are usually hulled and then boiled, toasted or roasted and eaten as a snack. They are very rich in protein, vitamins and minerals, such as zinc, iron and magnesium, and the seeds also produce a good quality oil that has culinary and other uses. Pumpkin oil is rich in unsaturated fats, Omega-3 and vitamin E, all of which make this oil a useful source of dietary fats. In Cameroon, Zambia and other countries, the roasted seeds are ground into a paste and added to various dishes for taste and nutrition.

Medicinal Properties

Regular consumption of pumpkin leaves, flesh or seeds increases antioxidants in the body and contributes to a balanced, healthy diet. The highly nutritious pumpkin with its wide array of vitamins and minerals can play a key role in improving health and well-being.

Pumpkin seed has been reported as being helpful in urinary disorders including for men living with benign prostate problems. The seeds' high fibre content is also useful in managing cardiovascular conditions, such as high blood pressure, high cholesterol and diabetes. High levels of zinc and magnesium also benefit heart health. Fresh and dried pumpkin has a high fibre content, which can limit glucose absorption, helpful for people living with diabetes.

Pumpkin seed oil has long been used for nourishing and moisturising hair and skin, and recent research suggests that the oil actually stimulates hair growth. The oil has anti-inflammatory properties so is useful in massages for tired, aching muscles and joints. This rich, green oil can also help to lower cholesterol and increase immune function.

History/Lore

There have been and perhaps will continue to be debates about whether pumpkin was first domesticated in the Central America or on the South American mainland. Some of the oldest seeds of the ancestors of this species have been found in caves in Oaxaca, Mexico and elsewhere in Belize and other parts of the region. Pumpkins are said to be one of the oldest cultivated plants.

Some indigenous myths in Central America refer to pumpkin as an incarnated goddess who descended from the heavens along with maize and beans. This speaks to the importance of pumpkin as a food crop in pre-Columbian societies. The important role that beans and maize had – and still have – in the history and culture of the peoples of Central America is common knowledge, but the pumpkin's role as part of this very nutritious trio is overlooked.

Queen Nanny of the Maroons is the only female Jamaica National Hero and played a vital role in the wars of resistance against slavery in the 18th century. She led the Windward Maroons in the rugged mountainous terrain of Portland against the British forces and defeated them. However, they were still able to burn the Maroon's villages and crops from time to time in revenge. Add to this seasonal hurricanes and drought and despite Nanny's success against the British forces, her people were facing starvation. Nanny was being urged by many to surrender to the British so that at least her people could get food, and she found the choice a very difficult one.

One night as she sought an answer to her dilemma, she was visited by her ancestors in a vision. They told her not to give up the struggle and to plant lots of pumpkin seeds, as this would help to feed her people. When Nanny awoke, she found some pumpkin seeds beside her, which she planted as directed by the ancestors.

These pumpkins helped to sustain the Maroons during their struggle, and today there is still a place called 'Pumpkin Hill' in the Maroon Lands in Portland. Given the versatility and nutritional value of this plant, it is unsurprising that pumpkin saved the Maroons back in the 18th century; what is surprising, however, is that it is not more widely used to address food and nutrition insecurity in the 21st century.

Nutrition Information

Part of Plant	Protein	Carbohydrates	Fats	Vitamins	Minerals	Fibre
Fruit Pulp	2g	12–15g	1g>	A, C, E, B1, B2, B3, B9	Ca, K, Mg, Fe, P, Zn, Mn	2g
Leaves	5g	5g	1g>	A, C, B1, B2, B3, B6, B9	Ca, Fe, P, Mn	3g
Seeds	25–35g	20–25g	40–50g	A, E, K, B1, B2, B3, B6, B9	K, P, Mg, Ca, Zn, Se	5g

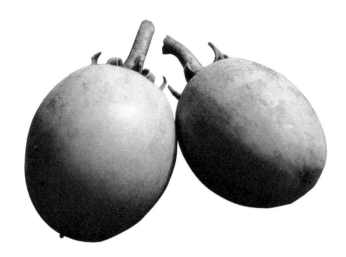

Shea

Local Names: *Karite; Butternut Tree; Lulu; Se; Taanga; Kareje; Sukpam; Ngu; Mai; Kolo*

Botanical Information: *Vitellaria paradoxa (Sapotaceae)*

The shea tree is native to the Southern Sahel region in Africa and is one of the most important trees across the swathe of Africa where it still grows. The savannah belt spreads south for about 300 km from Senegal, and then east for over 1,000 km across 15 different countries. This swathe has been the traditional home of the shea tree, which has played and continues to play a crucial role in the culinary, social, economic and cultural lives of the people in what is called the 'Shea Belt'.

One report estimated that there were more than 500 million shea trees across the wooded savannah of that belt. Shea trees do not grow outside of this geographical area and are the second most important oil crop after the palm nut tree in West Africa. The trees grow in stands and larger areas covering hundreds of hectares, or on smaller farms. Farmers are careful not to cut down the shea trees as they are highly valued; crops are therefore planted between the trees. In most of the dry savannah regions, shea are among the few trees that can survive in those soil and climatic conditions. Others include the African locust bean and baobab.

The tree is very attractive, reminiscent of European oak, growing up to 20 metres tall when mature, and about 1 metre in width, with a dense crown and many branches. The bark is dark, thick, cracked into squares like a crocodile's skin and is critical in protecting the tree from fires that occur from time to time. The bright, shiny green leaves of the shea tree

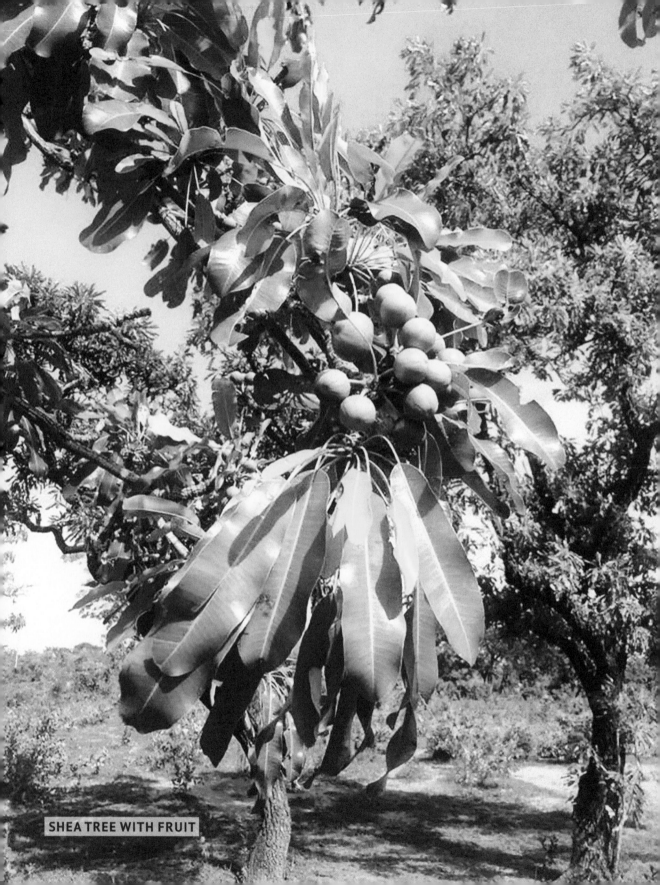

SHEA TREE WITH FRUIT

are quite tough and tend to bear at the end of the branches. The extensive root system is essential in helping the tree to survive seasonal and more prolonged droughts in the regions where it grows.

The flowers range in colour from creamy white to pale brown and do not bear fruit until 20–30 years after being planted. The trees can live for up to 400 years, but unfortunately do not fruit annually. Shea fruits resemble green plums and vary in size and shape: they are 3–6 cms and can be round or more elongated, growing at the end of a short stalk. The fruit pulp is thin, yellowish green, usually fairly sweet but can be quite tart, and softens as it ripens, with a texture similar to the European pear. Enclosed in the thin pulp is a proportionately large seed with a thin, brown shell that contains a dark-brown oval kernel.

Food Products

For more than 80 million people, shea butter is their primary cooking fat, and main source of dietary fats. It has been estimated that around 50% of the more than 1 million tonnes of shea nuts produced annually is exported, unprocessed, to Europe, Asia and the USA.

Shea fruits are collected, traditionally by women, and are eaten fresh as fruit or made into beverages, jams, jellies and fermented drinks. The fruits are usually available at the beginning of the annual rainy season and provide much-needed nutrients for rural populations as well as for those who buy the fruits at markets and street-side stalls in cities and larger towns. Shea is the source of income, however small, for many millions of poor households across the regions, where there are few crops of saleable value.

Shea fruits are rich in carbohydrates, vitamin C, calcium, phosphorous, magnesium and other minerals, but more importantly, for a fruit, they contain good amounts of protein. There have been recent initiatives to find ways to preserve the fruit pulp or incorporate it into more readily available products to treat nutritional deficiencies.

The main use of the shea fruit is, however, the nut or seed, from which the butter or fat is extracted. The traditional process for making shea butter has changed little for thousands of years and is laborious and time-consuming, but newer mechanical methods are now used in commercial production. The butter extracted by traditional methods is sold in containers or just in balls, rolls, in leaves or bottles, and despite being sold in markets in temperatures sometimes in the high 30s (Celsius), the butter does not melt.

Shea butter contains varying proportions of stearic acids (40–55%), which are unsaturated fats, oleic acids (35–45%), which are saturated fats and other fatty acids as well as non-fat constituents, such as sterols. The higher the proportion of the stearic acid content, the harder the consistency of the shea butter at ambient temperatures.

These properties have created a demand for shea beyond just being a cooking fat. The increased demand for shea outside of Africa is driven by commercial food and personal care products. Shea butter is similar to cocoa butter – another fat that is widely used in the above industries – but shea is cheaper to buy.

Other Uses

As mentioned above, shea butter is increasingly being used in the huge global beauty and personal care industry, due to its emollient and soothing properties. Shea is referred to as 'woman's gold' in the areas where it is produced. This is largely due to the contracts that some women's cooperatives have secured to supply high-end brands in Europe and other developed markets with shea butter. The quality and, more importantly, consistency in quality can vary across different areas and producers.

History/Lore

Archaeological excavations in Burkina Faso have unearthed ancient items that indicate shea butter has been produced and used in that region for thousands of years. West Africa was the first location for semi-domestication of shea trees, and they spread eastward across the savannah belt. There are key differences in the make-up of the shea butter produced by trees in Uganda compared to those in countries in West Africa. The oleic acid content is higher in shea nuts from Uganda in proportion to the stearic acid, and this is consistent, so they tend to produce shea oil there, which is being used increasingly in commercial production.

Shea samples in West Africa vary greatly in the stearic acid content, from 40–55%, but it is always proportionately higher than the oleic acids. Samples from the traditional heartland of production in Burkina Faso, the Mossi Plateau, consistently have the highest stearic acid content. Unsurprisingly, the shea butter from this region is renowned for its quality and is sought after by companies such as L'Occitane de Provence for use in their cosmetic and skincare products.

Another region famous for its shea butter production is Northern Ghana, which is geographically distant from the palm oil regions of Ghana. Shea butter is a common ingredient in the culinary culture of that region, and in fact the name of the largest city and capital of the region, Tamale, means 'place of the shea trees'. The Body Shop, another well-known international brand, has been sourcing shea butter for their products from a number of women's cooperatives around Tamale for more than thirty years. The company, like L'Occitane, has been recognised for the social and economic model they have, in terms of their contracts with the women producing the shea butter.

The United Nations Development Fund for Women (UNIFEM) played a very important role in the process, which led to the transformation of shea butter production in Burkina Faso and to women being empowered to demand the benefits of their labour.

The events which led to the formation of a cooperative – L'Association Songtaab-Yalgré – by Fatou Ouedraogo, a dynamic, Burkinabe woman, stemmed from unfair practices by some shea butter exporters, who did not pay the women who produced the butter well and treated them poorly overall.

The women's struggle is a case study in grassroots resistance, and the contract UNIFEM helped them negotiate has become a template for other women's groups that produce shea butter (or other products) for best practice in working with foreign business entities.

Nutrition Information

Part of Plant	Protein	Carbohydrates	Fats	Vitamins	Minerals	Fibre
Fruit Pulp	3–7g	45–60g	2g>	C, A	K, Fe, Ca, Mg, P, Zn	30–40g

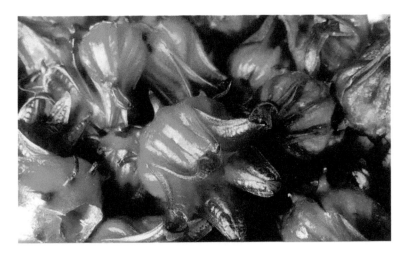

Sorrel

Local Names: *Roselle; Red Sorrel; Jamaica Sorrel; Bissap; Flor de Jamaica; Sour Tea; Karkade; Florida Cranberry; Rose d'Abyssine; Azeda de Guine; Ufuta; Zobo; Mesta; Zuring; Sobolo; Dah bleni*

Botanical Information: *Hibiscus sabdariffa (Malvaceae)*

Sorrel is thought to have been domesticated in the western regions of Sudan and spread eastward to the Arabian Peninsula and beyond to the Far East. Sudan remains one of the major producers of the plant, but sorrel is now grown from Senegal to East Africa, China, South and Southeast Asia, Central America and the Caribbean and in the Southern states of the USA.

It is an erect, annual shrub that grows up to 2.5 metres in height, with green and reddish stalks, which can be smooth or slightly hairy, with branched stems. The dark green leaves can have 3–5 pointed lobes and are 7–10 cms

long, and flowers can range in colour from pink to yellow and can be up to 12 cms wide. The distinctive red centre is the heart of the fruit, which takes the form of bright, fleshy, red calyces, which enclose small ovoid capsules (2–2.5 cms) that contain brown seeds. Sorrel prefers open spaces and can grow in temperatures of 18–35°C.

There are different types of sorrel, some edible, others that are grown for the fibrous stalks and some that do both. Of the edible types, red sorrel is the one that is most widely grown for its red calyces and leaves. The green

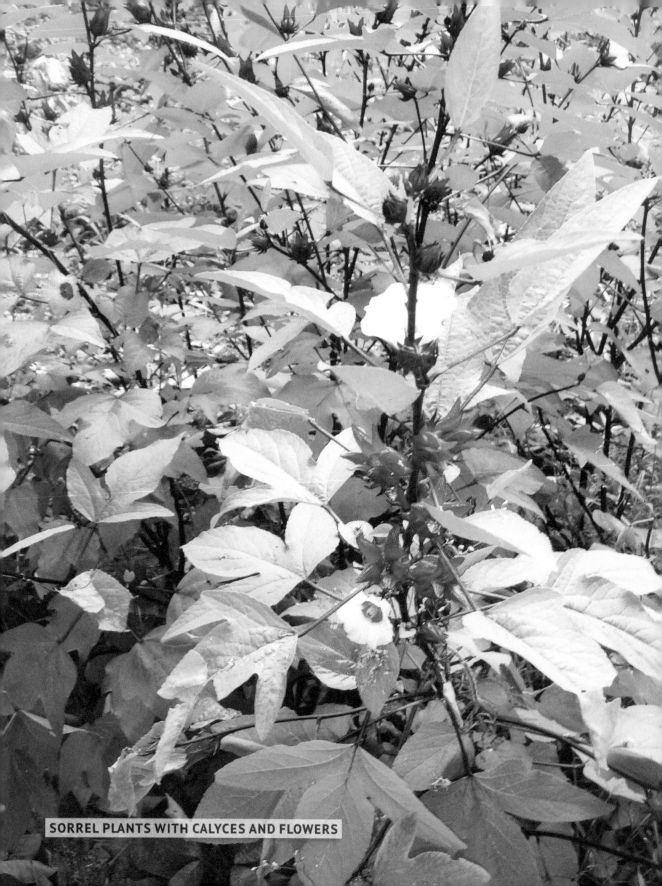
SORREL PLANTS WITH CALYCES AND FLOWERS

or the Middle East. Research has confirmed a measurable effect on blood pressure levels, but there are differing results as to how long this effect lasts. There is ongoing interest in the range of properties in the different parts of the sorrel plant that can be useful as nutraceuticals, especially in the management of chronic diseases.

Other Uses

Almost all parts of the sorrel plant are used for feeding poultry and livestock. The seeds are said to be a useful addition for chicken feed, and animals are often lucky to get abandoned plants where only the tender leaves were needed by the farmers or just the fruits. They also benefit from the residue of the oil extraction process.

The green variety is grown primarily for its leaves (food) and stalk (fibre). A family member, *H. cannabinus*, can grow 2–3 metres tall, and its stalks are harvested and processed for the fibre. While sorrel is not primarily cultivated for this purpose, today, the fibres from sorrel and its variants are being used alone and in combination with jute for bagging material and twine. The seed oil is used in making soap and other personal care products, with potential for even more varied applications.

History/Lore

Sorrel was taken to the New World from West Africa, where it had long been part of the traditional diet, and the light capsules containing the seeds would have easily been transported by the enslaved Africans. It was introduced into the Caribbean early in the 16th century, in particular on the island of Jamaica. The island's name has somehow become associated with the plant and the beverage: in Mexico and other parts of Latin America, sorrel is known as *Flor de Jamaica*, and the drink simply as *Jamaica*, pronounced as ha-MY-ka.

Sorrel was at one time grown in some areas more for the fibrous stalks than the succulent calyces. In the 1920s, Dutch colonial authorities began extensive cultivation of sorrel (*var altissima*) in the Dutch East Indies, now known as Indonesia, to produce fibre for sugar sack manufacturing. In India after the partition with Pakistan in 1947, there was a countrywide initiative to grow sorrel for fibre, as most of the jute production had been in Pakistan.

Nutrition Information

Part of Plant	Protein	Carbohydrates	Fats	Vitamins	Minerals	Fibre
Fruit/Calyx	2g	10g	1g>	C, B1, B2, B3, B6	Ca, Fe	2g
Leaves	3–4g	8g	1g>	A, C, B1, B2, B3	Ca, Fe, P	2g
Seeds	20–25g	25g	20g	C, B1, B2, B3	Ca, Fe, P, Mg, Zn	15g

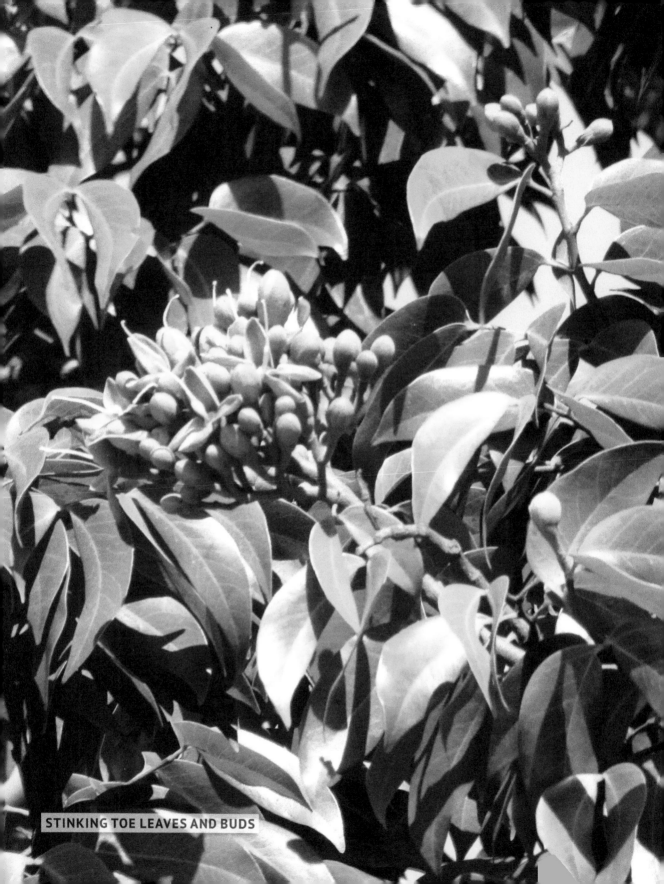

STINKING TOE LEAVES AND BUDS

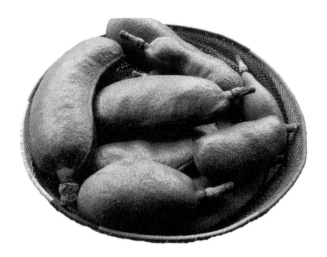

Stinking Toe

Local Names: *West Indian Locust; Jatoba; Brazilian Cherry; Guapinol; Algarrobo; Courbaril; Pois Confiture; Azucar Huayo; Rode Loksi; Kouhari; Jatai; Kerosene Tree*

Botanical Information: *Hymenaea courbaril (Fabaceae)*

Stinking toe is a large, evergreen tree with a dense, umbrella -shaped canopy and spreading branches. The tree is native to countries from southern Mexico through Central America to South America, except for the southern cone, as well as the Caribbean islands. The tree was also introduced into China, Sri Lanka, Indonesia and Malaysia in the 19th century. Stinking toe can grow in a wide range of soils and conditions, from tropical wet and dry lowlands up to 1,000 metres above sea level in wet and dry uplands. It can tolerate drought for a few months, but thrives where the annual rainfall is 1,500–3,000 mm.

Stinking toe tree grows slowly but can reach 30 metres or more in height and have a diameter of 1–2 metres. The smooth, grey to brown bark is up to 3 cms thick and when cut, exudes a resin. In fact, most parts of the tree contain some amount of resin, especially the roots. The shiny green leaves are distinct, as each leaf is formed from two leaves, matched like a couple. Creamy or white flowers occur in clusters and are pollinated by bats and bees. The fruit is oblong, varying in length from 5–15 cms and 3–5 cms in width, and the leathery pod looks like a giant toe, especially when it matures and turns from green to shades of brown.

The fruit is named not only for its looks but also for the smell, which can be described as pungent. The outer cover becomes tougher as it ripens and is quite hard to open. Once open, the 3–5 seeds are covered in a yellow to light-brown powder, which is fibrous in appearance and mealy in texture. Stinking toe pods can stay on the tree for up to seven months before falling to the ground. If the trees are fully grown, people wait to collect them beneath the tree, but smaller ones can be climbed or reached from the ground.

Food Products

Stinking toe can be eaten from the pod but is more often used to make a variety of food products. The fruit pulp is used to make various beverages, including fermented ones, and in Jamaica, stinking toe is combined with other ingredients to make a 'punch' that is reputed to be delicious, healthy and an aphrodisiac. Wherever the tree grows, there are local drinks and desserts made with the fruit.

In Brazil, where stinking toe is grown widely and goes by a multitude of names, the fruit pulp is sifted and stored and used as a flour. This can be added to porridges but is mainly combined with wheat, corn or cassava flour and made into 'broinhas', breads and other baked products. Stinking toe flour is similar in terms of protein content to wheat and corn but is higher than cassava so can improve the overall nutrition of these cereals.

Stinking toe is a rich source of carbohydrates and fibre and has vitamins A, B and C as well as minerals such as calcium, magnesium and iron. Its naturally low moisture content makes it useful for food security, as it has a long shelf life, especially when stored in sealed containers.

There has been increasing commercial usage of polysaccharides extracted from the seeds and fruits of the stinking toe. These are used in many food industry processes to improve the texture and taste of ice cream, baked goods and confectionery among others.

Medicinal Properties

Almost all parts of the stinking toe tree are considered to have healing or health-giving properties. As mentioned earlier, the fruit has a very high fibre content, which offers a host of benefits from digestive cleansing to management of blood sugar levels. Stinking toe also benefits from its high vitamin C content and other non-nutrient compounds that have significant antioxidant effects. High levels of beta-carotene contribute to improved eye health and reduce the likelihood of VAD. The presence of B vitamins offers protection against diseases such as beri-beri in an easily accessible form.

In parts of Central and South America, the bark of the stinking toe tree is reputed to be a cure-all, and many health conditions are believed to be improved by regular intake of bark extracts. In Brazil, there is a popular beverage, called jatoba, which is widely drunk as an energy drink and tonic.

When the tree is punctured, a sap called 'anime' is extracted, and this also has a reputation for the treatment of chest infections, urinary tract infections and other health problems. The resin is either burnt and inhaled to relieve asthma, and various local medicines are made using the resin or sap. The leaves are used for diabetes and fungal infections and the fruit can help to heal mouth ulcers.

Other Uses

Although stinking toe is regarded as a semi-wild tree, it is often cultivated for its wood, which is traded internationally as Brazilian cherry and is used to make hardwood floors and furniture. Charcoal is usually made with the leftovers of the lumber process or from smaller, irregular stock and branches. The resin, which is so popular for medicinal and other purposes, and bark are usually taken from trees that are destined for the lumber industry, to reduce debarking of fruit-producing trees.

The seeds and shell of the fruit are used to produce craft items. In Costa Rica, one side of the seed is sanded down, and miniature paintings are done and used as pendants. Stinking toe resin is used in the manufacture of varnishes, lacquers, sizing and paints, and polysaccharides from the seeds are used in the pharmaceutical and cosmetic industries.

History/Lore

Stinking toe is part of the Hymenaea genus, which was so named because of the distinctive feature of the leaves, that are made up of matching pairs of leaflets. Hymenaeus was the Greek God of weddings. All the hymenaea genus produce varying amounts of resin. There are reported to be 14 existing species

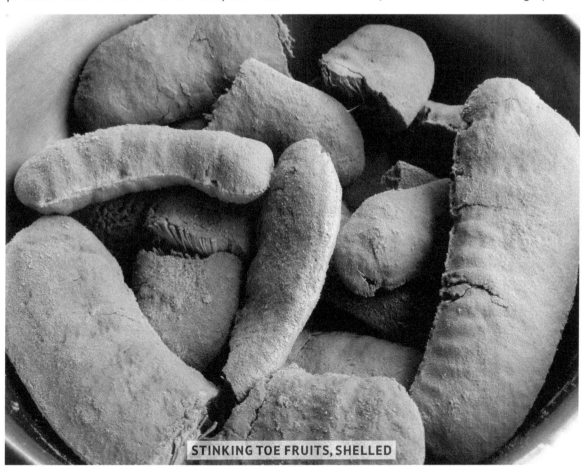

STINKING TOE FRUITS, SHELLED

of the genus, and all except one are native to the Americas. The exception is *H. verrucosa*, which is native to the coastal forests of East Africa and is the source of Zanzibar or East African copal.

One of the questions that has intrigued botanists is how these two similar trees are related, and at one time, *H. verrucosa* was assigned to a separate genus. However, advances in technology have made it possible to examine plant DNA more closely, and the tree has been reassigned to the hymenaea genus.

Amber has proven to be the key to unlocking some of the mystery because amber is essentially a polymerised form of the tree resin, a natural chemical process. However, that process takes millions of years. Scientists have analysed amber found in Mexico that contains leaves and other parts of a hymenaea species called *H. mexicana*, which is now extinct but is said to be related to *H. verrucosa*.

There are several theories as to how this might have occurred, including one that South America and Africa were in distant prehistory one super-continent called Gondwanaland. The separation of the continents may have left this particular species isolated in Africa, while the other species evolved in the Americas and the Caribbean.

The other theory is premised on the seed pod, with its unique characteristics, which could have been dispersed by ocean currents, some say from Africa to South America, others suggest the other direction. We may have to wait a little longer to solve the mystery of these prehistoric trees.

Nutrition Information

Part of Plant	Protein	Carbohydrates	Fats	Vitamins	Minerals	Fibre
Fruit Pulp	5.9g	75g	2–3g	A, C, B1, B2, B3	Ca, Mg, K, Zn, Fe	10–15g

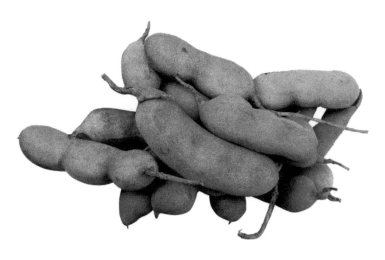

Tamarind

Local Names: *Indian Date; Tamarin; Tamr Hindi; Hemar; Dakhar; Tomi; Mkwaju; Dabe; Ajagbon; Tamarindo; Ambli; Ma-Khram*

Botanical Information: *Tamarindus indica (Fabaceae)*

Tamarind is said to have originated on the dry savannah of Africa from the coast of Senegal, to Central Africa, spreading eastward to the coastal parts of East Africa, from where it spread to the Indian subcontinent and beyond. Tamarind has adapted to growing in semi-arid as well as humid monsoonal conditions and now grows in more than 50 countries around the world.

Asia produces most of the tamarind that is traded internationally, and there are large areas being cultivated on a commercial scale, particularly in Thailand and the Philippines. Despite some demand for this crop, tamarind has remained an orphan crop in most countries in Africa and the Caribbean, where its potential to improve nutrition, increase rural development and conserve the environment remains largely unrecognised.

Tamarind is a tall, evergreen tree that can reach 10–20 metres in height depending on growing and other conditions. It has a sturdy girth, long, drooping branches, and its feathery, compound leaves form a dense canopy that can be up to 10 metres wide. The tree is slow growing and does not begin to fruit until 10–15 years after planting, but tamarind trees live for an average 50 years and there are trees that are more than 200 years old.

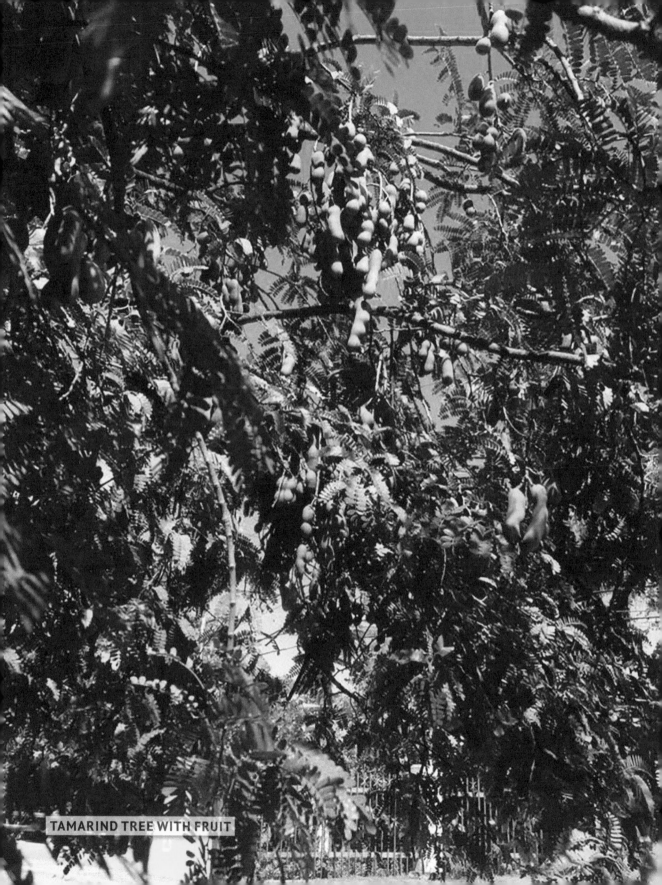

TAMARIND TREE WITH FRUIT

The flowers bear in clusters and are pale yellow, often with a pink undertone, and once the trees begin fruiting, they generally bear every other year. The fruit is a long, irregular-shaped pod, grey-green on the outside when immature, with pale-green flesh and white seeds. Tamarind pods can contain from 2–10 seeds; as the pods mature, the pulp enveloping the seeds becomes dark brown, sweeter and stickier, and the outside of the pod gets browner and more brittle. The mature seeds are dark brown to black and shiny with a tough seedcoat. If intact, the fruits can remain on the tree for up to six months after ripening, without loss of quality.

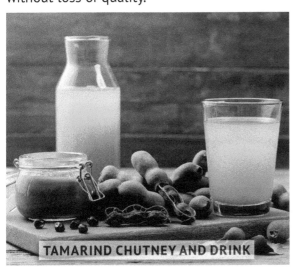
TAMARIND CHUTNEY AND DRINK

Food Products

The leaves, fruits and seeds of the tamarind can be used for food and nutrition, but the fruit pulp is the most widely used part. It is pulped and preserved in many ways and used to make various beverages, sauces and condiments. Tamarind is packed with or without seeds, salted or with sugar and kept in airtight containers for use. In the Sahel, the fruits are shelled, layered with sugar, sun-dried and pressed into cakes or balls and stored for future use. Every region or group has their own preferred way of preserving or processing tamarind.

Tamarind juice or nectar is enjoyed wherever available and is a key ingredient in the internationally known Worcestershire Sauce, in an award-winning pepper sauce from Jamaica called 'Pickapeppa', as well as being the 'secret' ingredient in many barbecue sauces. In traditional South Asian cookery, tamarind is included in curries, soups and delicacies. In countries like Mali, Burkina Faso and Niger, commercially produced tamarind drinks, some carbonated, rival more internationally known soft drink brands, and there is also a thriving trade in homemade versions of tamarind beverages and confections.

This fruit might not be as well-known as some others, but tamarind's many nutrients should make it more popular. The pulp has a relatively high protein content for a fruit, and it is also rich in B vitamins, notably a high percentage of thiamin and niacin. Although tamarind is known for its acidic flavour, it is not as high in vitamin C as its acidity would suggest. It does, however, have very high levels of calcium, iron and sugar.

Tamarind leaves are used in Africa and Asia as a vegetable, becoming higher in tannin as they age, so young, tender leaves are preferred. The leaves are either blanched in hot water and then sautéed with spices in oil or ground and mixed with spices and added to various dishes. They are rich in vitamins A and C and minerals such as calcium and potassium as well as useful amounts of protein. In parts of India and Southeast Asia, the young leaves are cleaned, dried and powdered for later use, providing additional nutrients for those who need them.

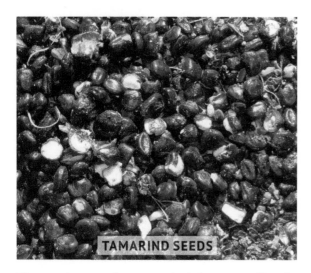
TAMARIND SEEDS

The real story for tamarind, however, lies in its underutilised potential as a nutritional powerhouse. The seeds are regularly discarded as part of the pulping process, sometimes being used to make feed for livestock. Tamarind seeds have to be de-hulled before use, due to the anti-nutrients in the seedcoats, which incidentally have their own properties and add to the potential of these humble seeds.

Tamarind seed kernels are rich in protein, carbohydrates and oil, with a well-balanced amino acid profile and high levels of calcium, potassium and phosphorous. They compare favourably to soya beans and other legumes, and the roasted seeds are said to taste like groundnuts. The seeds produce a flour which can be mixed with wheat and other flours to make baked goods. Oil can be extracted from this flour, and with some further refinement, tamarind seed oil, which has both saturated and unsaturated fats, could be used more widely for culinary purposes. It does, however, have lots of other applications and uses.

The tamarind seed is a source of a polysaccharide, xyloglucan, which is used extensively in food processing and in other industries. This and other seed extracts are used as emulsifying and gelling agents in the food-processing industry.

Medicinal Properties

Most parts of the tamarind tree have long been used for medicinal purposes in Africa, China, Asia and the Americas. The high mucilage content has been the main reason for the fruit pulp's traditional use in cases of constipation and bronchial problems. Tamarind is popularly believed to be helpful in losing weight and improving cardiovascular health.

The leaves are used internally and externally for joint and other inflammatory conditions and for skin problems such as heat rash. The seed including seedcoat can be ground and made into extracts which have beneficial properties for the skin.

Other Uses

One of the main uses of tamarind is as an invaluable shade tree in places that desperately need it. The tree's extensive roots system performs a key role in reducing soil erosion, and the foliage, which usually shed only in drought conditions, helps to enrich the soil when the leaves do fall. Due to the wide canopy and dense foliage, little grows under or near the tamarind tree, and this helps to reduce the spread of ground fires in the dry savannah. The trees are sometimes planted in stands as firebreaks, both for the lack of undergrowth as well as the tamarind tree's natural features, which help it to survive these sporadic or seasonal fires.

The seed oil can be used to make soaps, moisturisers, lotions and other personal care products, due to its emollient and hydrating properties. Other seed extracts, including hyaluronic acid and other fruit acids, are reputed to be effective in reducing fine lines and wrinkles.

Tamarind seed oil is also used in the production of paints, and the seedcoat which is high in tannin, is used in textile dyeing and paper sizing. Xyloglucan and other extracts are used widely in the pharmaceutical industry.

History/Lore

Botanical names generally reflect features of the particular plant, its relation to something else in nature or honour a botanist or plant enthusiast. Sometimes it is named to recall the location of its origin or where it was first discovered. *Tamarindus indica* is an instance where inaccurate information has been doubled down on in the naming of this tree.

It is said that the name tamarind is from the Arabic *Tamar al hindi* or Indian Date. The fruit is mentioned in ancient Sanskrit text, and most people in the West were likely introduced to this fruit via the Indian subcontinent. It has been clearly established for some time now that the tree originated in Africa, and genetic comparisons have confirmed that the tree spread eastward and was carried to the subcontinent by Arab traders from the east coast of Africa, where there has been long-standing trade relations between those regions. The second part of the name – *indica* – means Indian, so the misnomer has been squared. It is still not too late for a name change, and sometime in the future it might be called *Tamarindus africana*.

In some places where the tamarind tree grows, it has given rise to some strange beliefs, especially because nothing grows beneath it. Another feature that has given rise to myths about the tree is that the leaves go to sleep at night. If seen at night, they are folded. It is a feature not dissimilar to the actions of the shame plant (*Mimosa pudica*), which happens to be a distant relative of the same Fabaceae family.

Dakar is the capital city of the West African country, Senegal, and is also the Wolof name for the tamarind, suggesting that there must have been many tamarind trees in that area at some point in the past. Tamarind trees still grow across most parts of Senegal and if you are ever there, you can get a cool glass of *dakhar* juice, which is made out of tamarind.

Nutrition Information

Part of Plant	Protein	Carbohydrates	Fats	Vitamins	Minerals	Fibre
Fruit Pulp	3–5g	60g	1g>	B1, B2, B3, B5, B6, B9	K, Ca, Fe, Mg, P, Se, Zn	5g
Seed Kernel	18–25g	65g	6g	B1, B2, B3	P, Mg, Ca, K, Fe, Zn, Mn	4g
Leaves (Dried)	10–15g	70g	3g>	A, C	Ca, Fe, Zn, K	

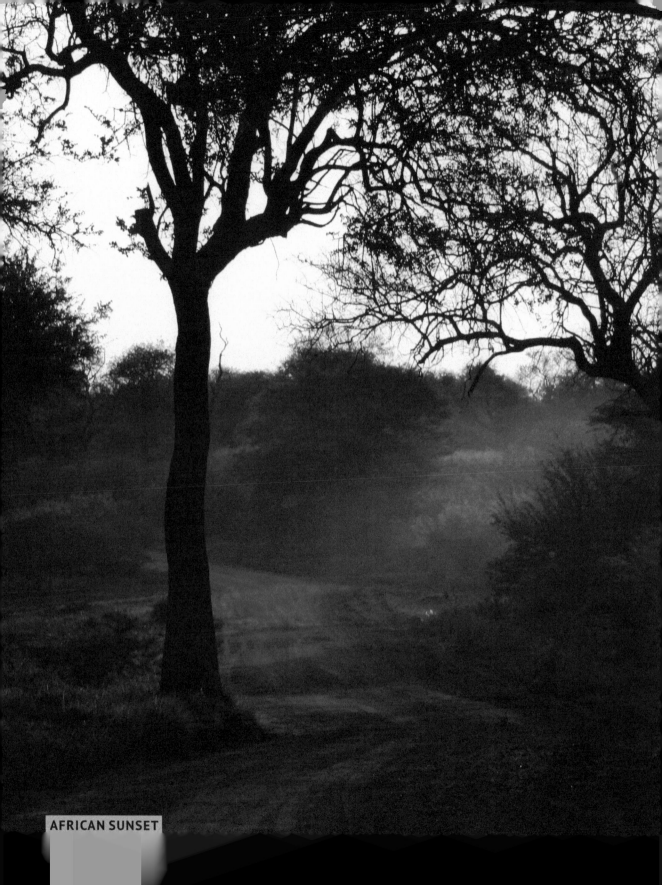

AFRICAN SUNSET

GLOSSARY

AGRA	Alliance for a Green Revolution in Africa
Biodiversity	The variety of living species (animal, plant, bacteria etc.)
EU	European Union
Food Security	The availability of food and access to it
Functional Food	Food that provides health benefits as well as nutrients
GGW	The Great Green Wall
G8	Informal bloc of seven industrial democracies plus Russia
GMO	Genetically modified organism
Indigenous	Originating in a particular place; native
Kwashiorkor	Protein energy deficiency disorder, usually in children
Marasmus	Deficiency in energy intake, especially carbohydrates
Maroons	Runaway Africans and their descendants in the Americas
MEP	Member of the European Parliament
Musculo-skeletal	Relating to muscles and joints
MM	Micronutrient malnutrition
NAFSN	New Alliance for Food Security and Nutrition in Africa
New World	Countries in the Americas
NCDs	Non-communicable diseases (non-infectious diseases)
NGO	Non-governmental organisations
Obesogenic	Contributing to obesity
PEM	Protein energy malnutrition
SDGs	Sustainable development goals
SOFI	State of Food Insecurity in the World
WHO	World Health Organisation

METRIC MEASURES

100 grams (g)	=	3.5 ounces
1 kilogram (kg)	=	2.2 pounds
100 millimetres (mm)	=	3.94 inches
2.54 centimetres (cms)	=	1 inch
1 metre (m)	=	39.37 inches
100 kilometres (kms)	=	62.13 miles
1 hectare	=	2.47 acres
1 litre	=	1.1 quart

NUTRITION – KEY FACTS

The Role of Nutrients in Our Bodies

The main purpose of this book is to provide information on crops that can contribute to food security, improved nutrition, environmental sustainability and rural social and economic development in some of the world's most vulnerable countries.

Throughout the book, I have stressed the importance of having access to food that is good quality, adequate, regular and nutritious. If the food we consume does not provide us with the range of nutrients that we need, some form of malnutrition will occur, and this in turn will affect our ability to function and grow.

It is amazing how little we learn about nutrition and the role of nutrients in our life as part of our education. Something so fundamental to our existence is unknown to many of us, and when we do get information, it is often dense and disconnected. Even in so-called developed countries, people are advised to read the labels on goods they buy, usually in supermarkets, to find out the nutritional value of the contents. Most would admit to being unsure of what all the numbers and percentages really mean, and the scientific terms only add to the lack of understanding. In most countries, where food is not always sold in original packaging or is sold in its natural form, there are no nutrition labels.

Food consumption, globally, continues to be driven by preference, practice, prices and presence (availability). Over time, people from different cultures have by chance or design come up with dishes that are not only delicious but also nutritious. Unfortunately, there are also many examples where the preferred food choices do not contribute to improving overall nutrition. Knowledge of what is in the food we eat can help us make informed choices when purchasing foodstuff to ensure that we get what is best for our bodies within our respective budgets.

Nutrients

Nutrients are divided into two major categories: **macronutrients** and **micronutrients.**

Macronutrients are those that the body needs regularly in large amounts. These are protein, carbohydrates and fats, and the primary role of these macronutrients is to provide the body with energy (calories).

Micronutrients are those that the body needs in smaller amounts. They include both water- and fat-soluble vitamins and a range of minerals.

Macronutrients

Carbohydrates

- Provide energy, particularly during high-intensity activity;
- Spare the use of proteins for energy;
- Provide fuel for the central nervous system (CNS);
- Break down fatty acids;
- Provide dietary fibre and natural sweeteners for foods.

Food Sources: whole grains, dairy products, fruits, vegetables.

Proteins

- Contribute to formation of tissue structure;
- Are involved in metabolic transport and hormone systems;
- Help to regulate metabolism;
- Maintain neutral environment in the body.

Food Sources: animal products, legumes, seeds, whole grains, nuts.

Fats

- Are an energy source and a reserve;
- Protect vital organs;
- Provide insulation within the body;
- Transport fat soluble vitamins.

Foods Sources: oils, nuts, seeds, dairy products, fish.

Micronutrients

Vitamins

Vitamin B1 – Thiamin

- Water-soluble vitamin, as are all of the B vitamins, which are needed to release energy in food;
- Essential in preventing beriberi disease;
- Keeps the nervous system healthy.

Food Sources: fortified cereals, whole grains, dried beans and peas, groundnuts, animal products, fresh and dried fruits.

Vitamin B2 – Riboflavin

- Needed to build and maintain eyes, skin and body tissues;
- Helps the body release energy from food.

Food Sources: whole grains, animal proteins, green and yellow vegetables, fortified foodstuff.

Vitamin B3 – Niacin or Nicotinic Acid

- Helps in modulating the metabolism;
- Plays a role in cell signals and DNA repair.

Food Sources: animal products, eggs, fish, greens, fortified foodstuff, whole grains.

Vitamin B5 – Pantothenic Acid

- Helps in making red blood cells that carry oxygen around the body.

Food Sources, cabbage family, beans, nuts, animal products, whole grains.

Vitamin B6 – Pyridoxine

- Helps in development of CNS;
- Involved in production of blood;
- Helps break down protein and glucose to produce energy for the body.

Food Sources: legumes, fruits, potatoes, yeast, nuts, whole grains, fish.

Vitamin B7 – Biotin

- Good for hair, skin, eye health and CNS;
- Helps to break down fat in the body;
- Is important during pregnancy for growth of baby.

Mainly made by the natural bacteria in the bowel; it is also found at very low levels in a wide range of foods.

Vitamin B9 – Folic Acid

- Helps build DNA and protein;
- Helps maintain intestinal tract;
- Aids in bone growth;
- Helps to reduce the risks of central neural tube defects in foetal development.

Food Sources: dark green, leafy vegetables, fortified cereals, wheatgerm, yeast.

Vitamin B12 – Cobalamin

- Keeps the body's blood cells and nervous system healthy;
- Helps to make DNA and also to prevent anaemia.

Food Sources: meat products, fish, fortified cereals, dairy products, eggs.

Vitamin A – Retinol

- Fat soluble vitamin that improves eye health;
- Improves skin elasticity and condition;
- Improves hair health.

Food Sources: animal products; the body makes vitamin A from foods that have carotene (sweet potato, mango, pumpkin, carrot); dark green leafy vegetables.

Vitamin C – Ascorbic Acid

- This is a water-soluble vitamin that plays a key role in improving the immune system;
- It helps to form growth hormones and is needed to help build strong bones, teeth and gums;
- Vitamin C has antioxidant properties.

Food Sources: most fruits and vegetables.

Vitamin D

- A fat-soluble vitamin that promotes strong teeth and bones;
- Can prevent rickets disease.

Food Sources: dairy products, fortified foods, fish oils, oily fish.

Produced by the body when exposed to sunlight.

Vitamin E

- Fat soluble vitamin that acts mainly as an anti-oxidant to prevent damage to cells and to enhance immune function;
- Helps to improve eye health and reduce the formation of clots in arteries.

Food Sources: plant-based oils, nuts, seeds, green, leafy vegetables.

Vitamin K

- Fat soluble vitamin, the main function of which is to aid blood clotting.

Food Sources: green, leafy vegetables.

Produced by bacteria in the large intestine.

Minerals (Chemical Symbol)

Calcium (Ca)

- The most abundant mineral in the body;
- Maintains teeth and bones, plays a role in maintaining communication between the brain and other parts of the body;
- It improves muscle movement and cardiovascular function;
- Vitamin D is needed to help the body to absorb calcium;
- Calcium can interfere with absorption of iron in the body.

Food Source: dairy products, fortified dairy alternatives, oily fish/bones, tofu, green leafy vegetables, whole grains, nuts, seeds, legumes.

Potassium (K)

- Helps the body to regulate fluid and the nerves to function;
- Important for heart health, helps prevent bone damage and kidney stones;
- Regulates muscle contractions, functions as an electrolyte and helps the body to remove excess sodium from the body;
- Reduces blood pressure and improves overall cardiovascular health.

Food Sources: dark-green leafy vegetables, sweet potato, mushroom, avocado pear, bananas, beans.

Iron (Fe)

- A major component of haemoglobin, which is a protein in red blood cells that carries oxygen from the lungs to all parts of the body;
- Important for brain development and growth in children;
- Aids production and function of different cells and hormones;
- Females aged from 15–50, need almost twice as much iron as men, and even more daily intake is necessary for pregnant and lactating women.

Food Sources: iron from food comes in two forms: heme and non-heme.

Heme iron is only found in meat, poultry and seafood. Non-heme is found in plant foods like whole grains, nuts, seeds, legumes, leafy green vegetables and iron-fortified foods.

Some foods inhibit the absorption of iron in the body, including those rich in calcium. It is best to eat non-heme iron foods with foods that are rich in vitamin C.

Zinc (Zn)

This a trace mineral, so although the body only requires small amounts, it is essential in order for about 100 enzymes to carry out vital chemical reactions, including growth of cells, building proteins, healing damaged tissue. Zinc is also involved with the sense of smell and taste and to support a healthy immune system.

Food Sources: whole grains, dairy products, fortified non-dairy milks, legumes.

Phosphorus (P)

This is the second most abundant mineral in the body. Phosphorus is essential in the creation of DNA and cell membranes. It is also key in the formation of teeth and bones, affects how the body uses carbohydrates and fats and is involved in the body's production of protein.

Food Sources: animal products, seafood, dairy products, seeds, nuts, dried fruit, whole grains.

Generally speaking, if you are meeting your protein and calcium requirements, your phosphorous levels should be adequate.

Magnesium (Mg)

This essential mineral is involved in many biochemical processes in the body. Magnesium plays a role in muscle and nerve function. It also helps to increase immune system function and overall bone strength.

Food Source: nuts (especially cashew and almond), legumes, soy products, whole grains, fruits, milk.

Manganese (Mn)

This might be called a trace mineral, but it is an essential one that is required for brain function and the CNS. Manganese also plays a role in many enzyme processes, and although the body does store some of the mineral, most of it has to come from the diet.

Food Sources: seeds, whole grains, legumes, nuts, tea, green, leafy vegetables.

Iodine (I)

This is another trace mineral that affects a wider range of body functions than obvious. Iodine is vital to ensure that thyroid hormones work properly. These hormones play an important role in metabolic function, immune response, bone health and the development of the CNS. Too much or too little can cause disorders and diseases, so having a balance is important. There are more than one billion people globally who experience iodine deficiency, with more than 300 million having thyroid problems.

Food Sources: iodised salt, seaweed, seafood.

Naturally occurring iodine is present to varying degrees in most foodstuff, including those from animal sources. The levels of iodine depend on the amount of iodine available in the soil where crops are cultivated or animals raised. As a rule of thumb, iodine levels decline the further you go from the ocean.

Selenium (Se)

This essential trace mineral is important for many bodily functions. It strengthens immune function, improves brain function, impacts fertility in both men and women and has antioxidant properties. Selenium also plays a role in thyroid metabolism and DNA synthesis.

Food Sources: brazil nuts; tuna and other large fish; brown rice and other whole grains.

Most foods have traces of selenium, but the amount depends on the level of the mineral present in the soil where food is produced.

Water

One of the most overlooked nutrients, water is vital to almost all the biochemical reactions in the body. It is worth remembering that water deficiency will cause more harm to the body more quickly than lack of any other nutrient. It is a lubricant for joints, moistens tissues such as those in the mouth, eyes and nose, helps to eliminate waste from the body and regulates body temperature. Water also helps to dissolve minerals and other nutrients to make them accessible to the body and carries nutrients and oxygen to cells.

Food Sources: water; most fresh fruits and vegetables contain water; cooked meals provide varying amounts of water; hot and cold beverages; small but significant amount made within the body.

Dietary Fibre

Dietary fibre is essentially the indigestible part of the plant foods we consume and is also called roughage. There is clear evidence that fibre plays an important role in our nutrition and overall health, and how it acts changes the nature and effects of gut bacteria. Gut ill-health is associated with a range of diseases, including inflammatory conditions, cardiovascular illnesses and some cancers.

We get our fibre either directly from plant sources such as grains, fruits, legumes, nuts, seeds and vegetables, or it can be derived from so-called functional fibre, which comes from substances added to food during processing.

There are two types of dietary fibre: soluble and insoluble. Soluble fibre absorbs water and forms a gel-like substance in the digestive tract. The main sources are from fruits, legumes and oat bran. Soluble fibre supports gut function, softens stools, slows rate of glucose absorption thus playing a key role in managing blood sugar and also reduces LDL or 'bad' cholesterol.

Insoluble fibre does not dissolve in water and comes from grain bran, nuts and vegetables. It adds bulk to stool, shortens gut transit, relieves constipation and improves colonic health. It also helps with weight management, prevention of type 2 diabetes and improved cardiovascular health.

Proteins

The role of proteins was summarised earlier, but it is important to take a closer look at the make-up of these key nutrients. Significant amounts of proteins are present in muscles, skin, bones, hormones, antibodies and enzymes, and they are involved in many processes within the body.

Proteins are made up of 20 amino acids, and when proteins are consumed, they are broken down and amino acids are left, which the body then uses to make more proteins that perform all the roles and functions they do. Amino acids are also a source of energy for the body.

Amino acids are classified into three groups: essential amino acids, non-essential amino acids and conditional amino acids.

There are nine essential amino acids, and these have to come from the food we consume: histidine, isoleucine, leucine, lysine, methionine, phenylalanine, threonine, tryptophan, valine.

Non-essential amino acids are produced by the body, even when our diet does not provide them: alanine, arginine, asparagine, aspartic acid, cysteine, glutamic acid, glutamine, glycine, proline, serine, tyrosine.

All but four of these, (alanine, asparagine, aspartic acid, glutamic acid) are also described as conditional amino acids, which means that they become 'essential' in times of illness and stress.

Only foods that provide all the essential amino acids are called complete proteins.

Food Sources: animal products, seafood, dairy products.

Incomplete proteins usually lack one or more essential amino acids.

Food Sources: legumes, peas, beans, whole grains, fruits, vegetables.

The role and make-up of proteins are of particular interest to people who have plant-based diets or consume a high proportion of these types of food. Nutritionists used to advise vegetarians and vegans that they should combine different foods from the incomplete proteins, such as rice with beans or wholemeal bread with peanut butter, in order to get complete proteins.

The current thinking is that it is more important to get the balance of essential amino acids over the course of the day. It is therefore necessary to get the amino acids from a variety of plant foods, as consuming one type of food will not provide adequate amounts of proteins to meet the body's needs.

Having a good mix of seeds, nuts and whole grains will normally provide sufficient protein, but there are still millions of people, mostly in the developing world, who experience a chronic lack of protein in their diet. Protein deficiency in children is of particular concern and leads to conditions such as kwashiorkor, marasmus and unacceptably high rates of stunted growth. In adults, low protein levels can cause hormone imbalance, loss of muscle mass and an increase in the severity of infections.

Recommended average daily intake for adults is 50 grams per day; however, this may need to be higher based on activity level, pregnancy or other health circumstances. Excessive protein intake can also result in health problems. It has been linked to a range of cardiovascular diseases, kidney damage, obesity and joint and tissue conditions, such as gout and arthritis.

Anti-nutrients

It might seem strange to be referring to 'anti-nutrients' in information on nutrition, but it is an aspect of nutrition that is often overlooked. All foods contain various substances that can provide humans with the different macro and micronutrients they require. Among the many compounds in food, some have the ability to be both beneficial and detrimental, depending on a few factors, which include stage of maturity consumed and condition of the item as well as the preparation and cooking method, if cooked.

Anti-nutrients are compounds or substances, of natural or synthetic origin, which interfere with the availability and absorption of nutrients in the body. In developed economies, diets are not usually impacted by these compounds, due to most protein in the diet coming from animal products. There are more food choices in developed economies, and most of the food that is consumed has been processed in some way.

The highest concentrations of anti-nutrients are found in grains, legumes, nuts, seeds, leaves and roots. This is more likely to affect people whose diets are plant-based such as vegetarian, vegan or raw food. It can also be an issue for the many millions of people who are food insecure and whose diets are primarily based on a limited range of grains, legumes, starchy tubers and vegetables. The recent SOFI Report estimates that in Sub-Saharan Africa, only 11% of the food consumed is from animal sources as compared to 20–30% in middle- and upper-income countries.

People have found methods which reduce or eliminate the most negative effects of these anti-nutrients, and some methods, in fact, increase the nutrients in the food. Many of the same compounds that are classified as anti-nutritional are used therapeutically for improving human health and often play a key role in the plant's own natural defence mechanism. The main issue is to raise awareness of these substances and to learn about the ways in which any impact they have might be mitigated.

Main Anti-nutrients

Lectins: wheat, quinoa, potatoes, nuts, especially almonds

Alpha-amylase Inhibitors: seeds

Protease Inhibitors: raw cereals, legumes, especially soya bean

Tannins: leaves, legumes, bark, tubers, grapes, green and black tea

Phytates: seeds, grains, nuts, legumes, cassava, potatoes, yam

Goitrogens: broccoli, cabbage, kale, cauliflower, quinoa, buckwheat

Oxalates: green, leafy vegetables, berries, beans, cassava, cocoyams, grains

Saponins: tomatoes, egg plant, potatoes, legumes

Trypsin Inhibitors: chickpeas, mung beans, kidney beans

Methods for Reducing/Eliminating Anti-nutrients

Soaking

Soaking in a solution of water, sodium bicarbonate and salt for periods of 12, 24, 48 hours or more and discarding the water can help to reduce the amount of particular anti-nutrients.

Fermentation

Many seeds, and grains can be fermented before use by using *L. acidophilus* or some other bacteria as a starter. This should be done at minimum of 37°C for at least 24 hours. This process should result in a reduction in anti-nutrients and an increase in protein and other nutrients.

Sprouting (Germination)

Sprouting of seeds, legumes and grains is one of the most effective methods of reducing or eliminating anti-nutrients and increasing the nutritional content.

Malting

Grains, usually, are sprouted, dried and then used. This process changes the chemistry of the grain and gives it the nutty, distinctive flavour that malted grains have.

Heating

A number of methods can be included under the umbrella term 'heating'. Typically, this is done by some form of cooking: boiling, frying, roasting, baking or exposure to some form of heat that changes the state of the food.

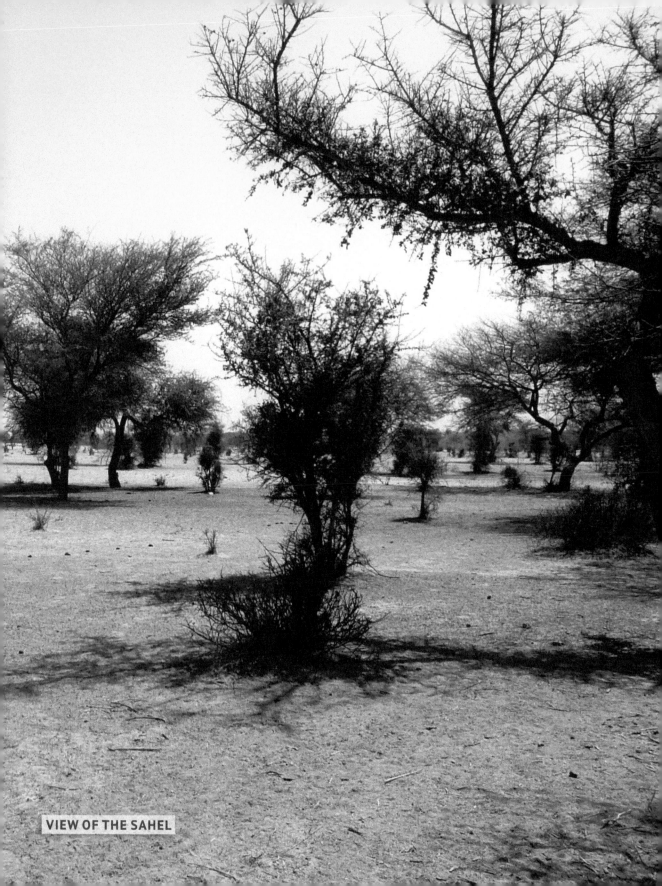

VIEW OF THE SAHEL

INFORMATION ON FOCUS REGIONS

The West African Sahel

The Sahel is a swathe of five million square kilometres of land that stretches from Northern Senegal to the Red Sea coast of Eritrea, between the Sahara Desert and the savannah and tropical lands to the south (see map: p. 134). The weather in the Sahel is characterised by long, dry periods, short, irregular periods of rainfall and high temperatures, which are rising 1.5 times faster than the global average. It is estimated that 80% of farmland in the Sahel can be classified as 'degraded', and the region has been described as 'a canary in a coal mine', indicating that what is happening there in terms of climate change is a foretaste of what is to come in other vulnerable parts of the world.

As a result of the ongoing desertification of the Sahel, there have been a number of initiatives to halt the encroachment of the Sahara Desert, regenerate the region's environment and increase agricultural and livestock production to improve the food security of the population. One of the biggest is The Great Green Wall (GGW) Project, which began in 2007, funded primarily by the African Union, individual governments in the participating countries and international funding agencies. The initial aim was to plant a wall of trees from Senegal to Djibouti, 15 kilometres wide, which would help to 're-green' the Sahel, resist the march of the desert, improve the environment and boost development in the region.

From the outset, experts and activists expressed doubts about the viability of the project or the likelihood that it would achieve its aims. Unfortunately, many of their concerns have been borne out, with large areas of planted trees dying due to neglect and water shortage. What has proven successful, however, has been efforts by small-scale farmers in countries like Senegal, Burkina Faso, Mali and Niger, who have used traditional, indigenous land use technologies to regenerate parts of the Sahel. As some critics have pointed out, there is less of a green wall and more of a mosaic of greening across the region.

Environmental challenges, including climate change, have brought about widespread changes in traditional relationships between herders and farmers. These once-symbiotic relationships have now turned into conflicts over scarce resources, further exacerbated by external players, who are capitalising on the desperate conditions there, particularly those of the youths in the region. Herders belong predominantly to nomadic and semi-nomadic groups like the Tuareg and Fulani among others.

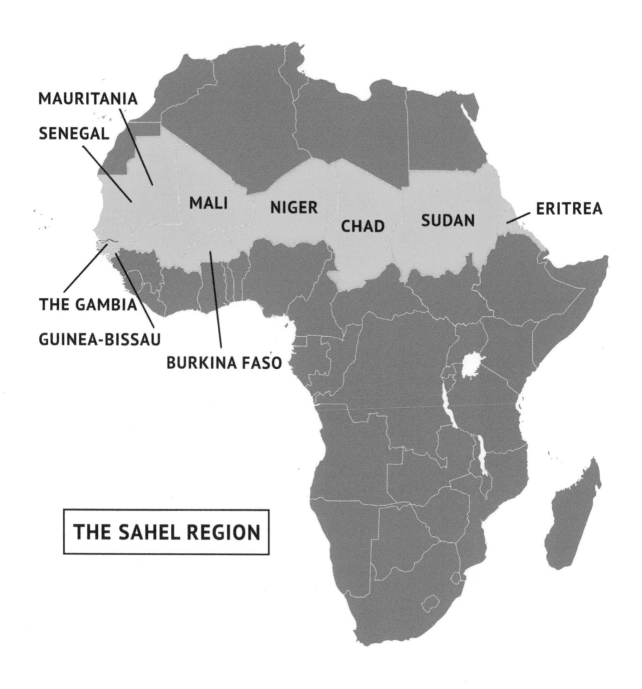

MAURITANIA

SENEGAL

MALI

NIGER

CHAD

SUDAN

ERITREA

THE GAMBIA

GUINEA-BISSAU

BURKINA FASO

THE SAHEL REGION

Because the Sahel is not defined by borders, it can be difficult to get data specific to the geographical area, so data are taken from the countries that fall inside the zone. For the purposes of this book, the focus is primarily on the West African Sahel, which includes countries such as Senegal, Mali, Burkina Faso, Niger, The Gambia and Chad. This region has a relatively high population, estimated at around 85–100 million people, a number which is expected to almost double by 2050.

Most of the countries in the Western Sahel have similar socioeconomic features, which contribute to the convergence of multidimensional challenges. These include poor existing infrastructure, fragile governance systems and high rates of unemployment and poverty, particularly among women and youths. For the most part, education and health systems fail to meet the needs of their rapidly growing populations, with the majority of the population (65%) being under 25 years.

Over recent decades, there has been an increase in urbanisation in the Sahel, driven by the failure of traditional occupations to provide an adequate standard of living. Many towns in the Sahel and neighbouring regions have developed rapidly with internal migration from rural areas no longer able to support traditional lifestyles. Most of the economic activities in these towns and cities can be described as informal. For most young people, who have become increasingly exposed to new technologies and media, their aspirations have been transformed, and they are no longer satisfied with the limited opportunities available to them.

Within the Economic Community of West African States (ECOWAS), citizens of the fifteen member countries have the right to travel, work and reside within the region. Generally speaking, people within the community are very mobile, but language, financial and other constraints prevent mass movement of the most needy, who therefore cannot access these opportunities. For those who succeed in migrating either to the coastal cities of ECOWAS countries or to Europe and beyond, their remittances play a key role in the social and economic development of the Sahel.

The Sahel is not only one of the main migrant routes to the Mediterranean region and beyond but also a source of migrants. Many of them have become 'climate change refugees', and the youth who fail to make it out easily fall prey to the overtures of religious and other ideological extremists, who recruit them for more nefarious and dangerous activities. Some of these same young men then become involved in the ongoing insurgencies across the Western Sahel involving any number of armed groups, which has led to increasing deaths and destruction in the region.

These civil conflicts have resulted in the internal displacement of large numbers of people. Farmers, who already faced many challenges, have had to flee from their land for security reasons; crops have been abandoned as whole villages have fled from violence. All this has made an already desperate situation turn into a humanitarian crisis. A perfect storm of climate change and civil conflicts have left more than five million displaced either internally or in neighbouring countries. Over 33 million people are now estimated to be food insecure in the West African Sahel.

Prior to the spread of civil conflicts in the region, most of the food consumed (80%) there, such as cereals, oilseeds, legumes, roots and tubers, had been traditionally produced across the Sahel and neighbouring regions. Despite the land degradation, the potential for agricultural self-sufficiency still exists. If the violence and threats of violence can be reduced or better eliminated, despite the many challenges, the farmers could be supported to provide for their families and communities.

Food insecurity leads inevitably to malnutrition, which in turn contributes to a range of health conditions, especially for young children and women. Countries in the Sahel have long had high rates of infant and maternal deaths, due in large part to high levels of pregnancies, poor diets and inadequate health services. The current situation has only made these conditions worse.

Inadequacies in the supply and availability of potable water also play a key role in poor sanitation, and there are high rates of infectious diseases, such as cholera, diarrhoea and various water-borne diseases. With so many people being internally displaced and living in overcrowded camps, conditions are rife for increased rates of infectious diseases. The current COVID-19 pandemic will only add to the disease burden among populations in the Sahel.

In the millennia prior to the arrival of Europeans in Africa, the Sahel was home to some of the greatest African kingdoms and empires in history. These include the Empires of Ghana, Mali, Songhay and Kanem-Bornu, which were recorded as thriving, well-organised states, and included centres of learning such as those in Timbuktu. The people who currently occupy the Sahel region will have to revisit the history of their ancestors, rediscover the crops that sustained them over time and develop strategies to survive the current and future challenges they face.

The Caribbean Region

The Caribbean region includes the islands in the Caribbean Sea as well as countries with a Caribbean coastline. For the purpose of this book, the focus will be on these islands and three countries on the Central and South American mainland: Belize, Guyana and Suriname, whose populations identify historically and culturally with the Caribbean region.

The Caribbean Sea lies between North and South America, covering more than 2.75 million square kilometres (see map: pp. 138–9). It is a diverse region, with differences in size, geography, population, political status and systems, culture, and levels of social and economic development. Languages in the region include French, Spanish, English, Dutch and various dialects that are a mixture of any of these with African, Asian and indigenous languages.

Most of the islands and territories in the region were captured during the period of European 'discovery' and land grabbing, and they were primarily established as plantation economies for export to the colonial powers. The history of this region has been characterised by violence, oppression, resistance and episodes of liberation. The Caribbean region has been populated by waves of migrants, enslaved, indentured and voluntary, and migration in all its manifestations continues to be a key issue in the region.

Despite the differences between the countries in the region, they share some common characteristics and challenges to a lesser or greater degree. The Caribbean region is the most indebted region in the world, with average debt to GDP ratios in excess of 70%. These high levels of national indebtedness are reflected in high rates of youth unemployment, widespread inequalities and crime. The region also experiences high energy costs, susceptibility to external shocks, natural disasters and environmental issues.

Many of these problems are obscured by the beautiful, picturesque landscapes of the Caribbean and some of the outward trappings of development, either as efforts to attract tourists or the result of remittances from nationals living or working overseas.

Complex patterns of migration contribute both positively and negatively to overall economic development, but they have also led to social and cultural issues which have had many negative impacts. The Caribbean is a region of origin, transit and intraregional migration. The region also experiences significant return migration, both voluntary and as a result of deportation, the latter posing a range of challenges for the deportees and their reintegration into local communities.

The Caribbean is a transit hub for the trafficking of illegal drugs, mostly from South America, people-smuggling as well as the smuggling of arms and ammunitions. Such activities have led to increases in crime and violence, carried out for the most part by ever-growing numbers of gangs in countries in the region.

Caribbean islands are in the path of seasonal hurricanes, which have become progressively more destructive in recent years. Interestingly, the majority of the Category 3, 4 and 5 hurricanes (85%) are reported to begin life near the Cape Verde Islands, off the coast of Western Africa. Each year, in anticipation of the coming season, individuals and governments have to spend considerable amounts of money for what is termed 'preparedness'.

Hurricanes and severe storms can wreak havoc on already fragile infrastructures, and the potential for damage and destruction on islands battered by a hurricane is growing with each season. As in most areas of life, the people who are more likely to be negatively impacted are those who are most ill-prepared due to their already low-income levels.

Apart from hurricanes, the Caribbean region is affected by droughts, floods and earthquakes, with hundreds of relatively small quakes each year. Experts predict that there could be a major quake in the region in the near future, similar to the one that devastated Haiti in 2010. Estimates of the number killed in that earthquake ranges between 100,000 and 220,000 people, with damage estimated at $5–7 billion.

The country was hit in 2016 by Matthew, a Category 4 hurricane, which caused widespread damage to infrastructure and agriculture of more than $1.9 billion and left almost 1,000 residents dead. Haiti still struggles with the effects of those natural disasters, and the island remains an outlier in the region, in terms of low levels of social and economic development.

Haiti has been afflicted in recent decades by environmental issues such as widespread deforestation, soil degradation and extreme weather events, all of which have a significant impact on efforts to increase agricultural production and food security. These same environmental issues are of concern to the middle-income countries in the Caribbean, particularly those that rely on tourism, including cruise shipping. The region is the most tourist reliant in the world with a product that is based primarily on the natural beauty and features of the islands. If the industry continues on its current path, damage to the natural environment will jeopardise the very product itself.

Tourism has provided an avenue for development for many of these islands which, because of their small size and other limitations, have fewer options. Unfortunately, in the wake of the activities and inputs that go to make up the tourism product, the environmental costs to these countries have become burdensome.

Coastal erosion, water scarcity, huge carbon footprints from energy use and the growing challenge of waste management are among the environmental challenges faced by tourism in the Caribbean. Small island states do not have the capacity or land space to cope and do not have the economies of scale to carry out effective and efficient recycling. Some islands are literally being choked by garbage, especially by the ubiquitous single-use plastic bags. However, danger also rests in waste materials that contain toxic chemicals and which need careful and expert disposal or treatment.

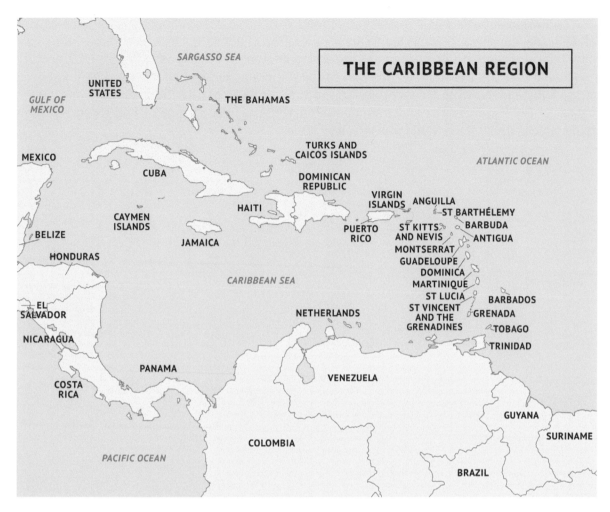

Scarcity of water and the quality of available water has also become an issue for the Caribbean region, as it grapples with competing pressures on water supplies. The tourism sector consumes huge amounts of fresh water, including supplying cruise ships that ply their trade in the region. Agriculture also requires water, and changes in weather patterns, below-average rainfall and more frequent and prolonged droughts are having an impact on productivity. This in turn hampers efforts to improve food security and nutrition.

Currently food insecurity in the Caribbean region is not as widespread as in other regions and is related to poverty and inequalities, with some countries and groups within states more vulnerable than others. Rates of undernourishment, although still present, especially in Haiti, are relatively low but expected to rise. There are, however, higher levels of obesity than the global average, with some islands such as Barbados having rates as high as 36% and, worryingly, increasing rates among children. The Caribbean region also has some of the highest prevalence of diet- and lifestyle-related non-communicable diseases (NCDs) such as diabetes, high blood pressure and heart disease, which account for most deaths among those aged 35–70.

The Caribbean imports a high proportion of food, with some islands importing as much as 80% of what they consume. This has led to the proliferation of unhealthy processed foods, which are high in fats, sugar and salt. Even more concerning are the data in the SOFI Report (2020) which concluded that the cost of a healthy diet in the Caribbean is three times the spending power of those living below the poverty line. If opportunities to access a healthy diet are beyond the means of significant sections of the population, there is little chance of improving nutrition, reducing obesity or improving food security.

RECIPES

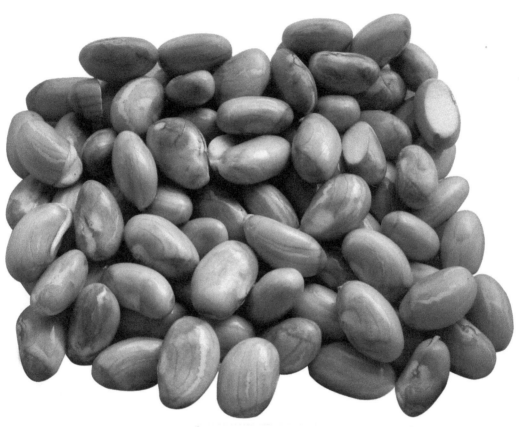

JACKFRUIT SEEDS

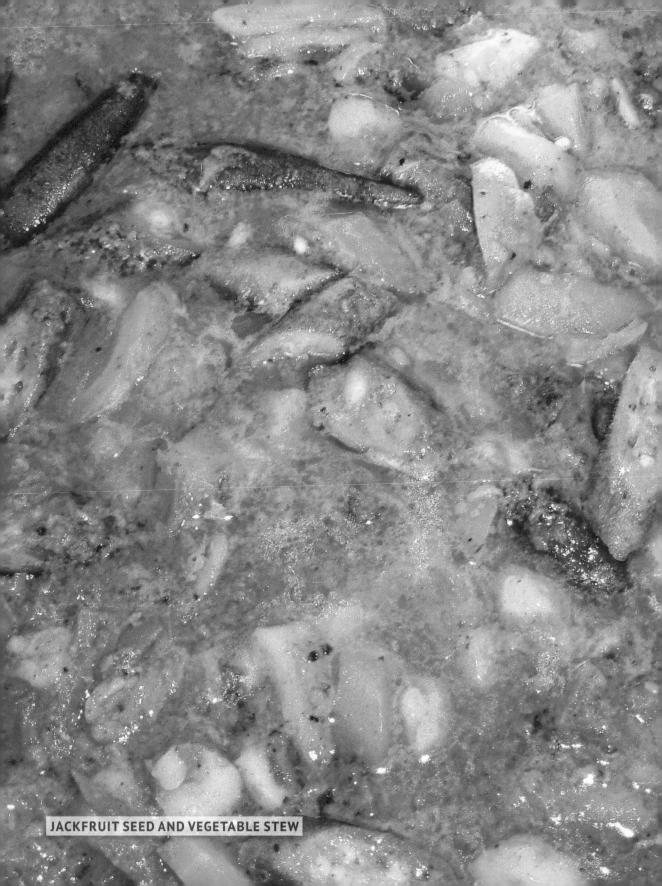

JACKFRUIT SEED AND VEGETABLE STEW

Jackfruit Seed and Vegetable Stew

Ingredients

100g	jackfruit seeds
150g	pumpkin
6	medium okras
1	large onion
2	medium tomatoes
4	cloves garlic
1	hot pepper
2 tbsp	oil
1 tsp	salt

Favourite spices and herbs

Preparation

Wash jackfruit seeds, cover with water, add half teaspoon salt and boil until fork-tender.

Discard water, rinse with cold water and remove the outer skin of the seeds. These can be left as is, sliced or mashed and set aside.

Heat oil gently in a sauce or fry pan, add chopped onions, garlic and hot pepper. Stirring as necessary, add spices and chopped tomatoes. Cover and leave for 10 minutes on low flame. Add half teaspoon salt and the jackfruit seeds and stir before covering.

Wash, peel, dice/slice pumpkin and add to pan. Cover with 200 ml water or vegetable stock and leave to simmer for 15mins. Add sliced or whole okras and cook for 5 more minutes before removing from heat.

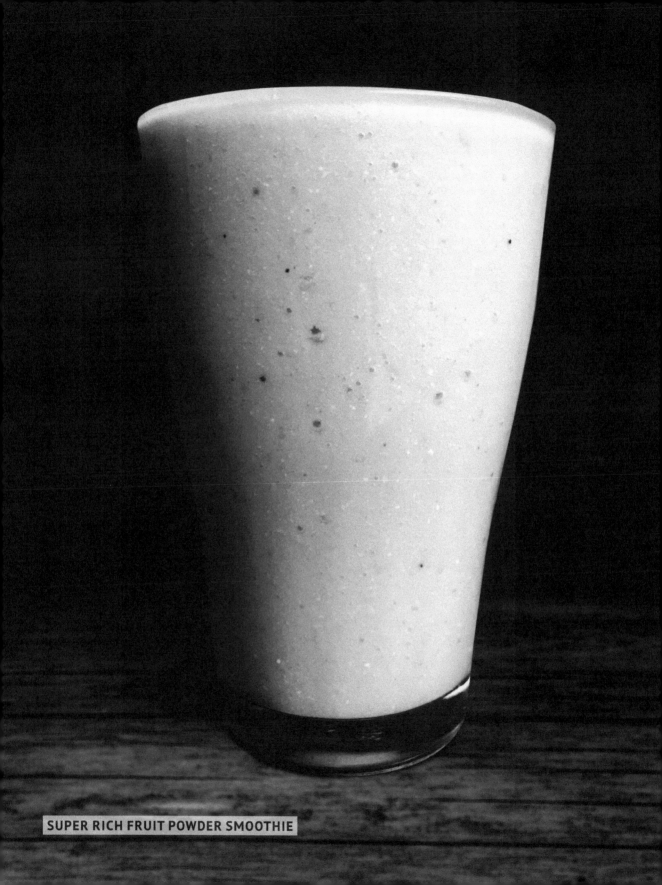

SUPER RICH FRUIT POWDER SMOOTHIE

Super Rich Fruit Powder Smoothie

Ingredients

50g	groundnut (peanut)
25g	stinking toe powder
25g	african locust bean powder
20g	baobab powder
400ml	plant milk (coconut, soy/almond/bambara bean)
2	bananas
1	small papaya

Add spices to taste

Method

Grind/blend groundnut and add the fruit powders. Add bananas, papaya, spices and milk. Blend together, chill, serve and full-joy.

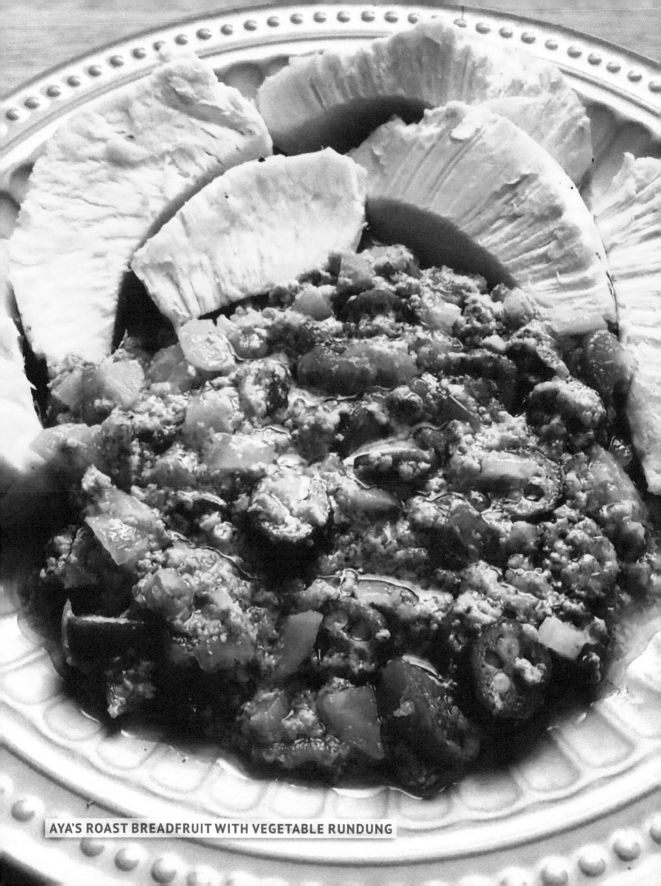

AYA'S ROAST BREADFRUIT WITH VEGETABLE RUNDUNG

Aya's Roast Breadfruit with Vegetable Rundung

Ingredients

1	breadfruit (firm, mature, unripe)
2	medium coconuts (blended) or 2 cups coconut cream
2	onions
2–3	tomatoes
1	carrot
3	okras

garlic, pepper, turmeric, salt, pimento berries to taste

Method

Roast Breadfruit

Place breadfruit on a charcoal stove or grill. Turn frequently to ensure even roasting (30–45 minutes) depending on size. Test by inserting knife through the heart of the fruit. When properly roasted, the knife should come out clean (similar to testing for a baked cake).

When thoroughly roasted, leave to cool before peeling the burnt skin. Slice and serve.

Vegetable Rundung

Put coconut milk or cream in a shallow saucepan and leave to boil until the 'custard' begins to form. Add chopped garlic, pepper and turmeric. When the custard thickens, add onions, tomatoes, carrot and okra. Leave pot uncovered throughout. Turn off heat after 5–10 minutes and allow to sit for a few more minutes before serving.

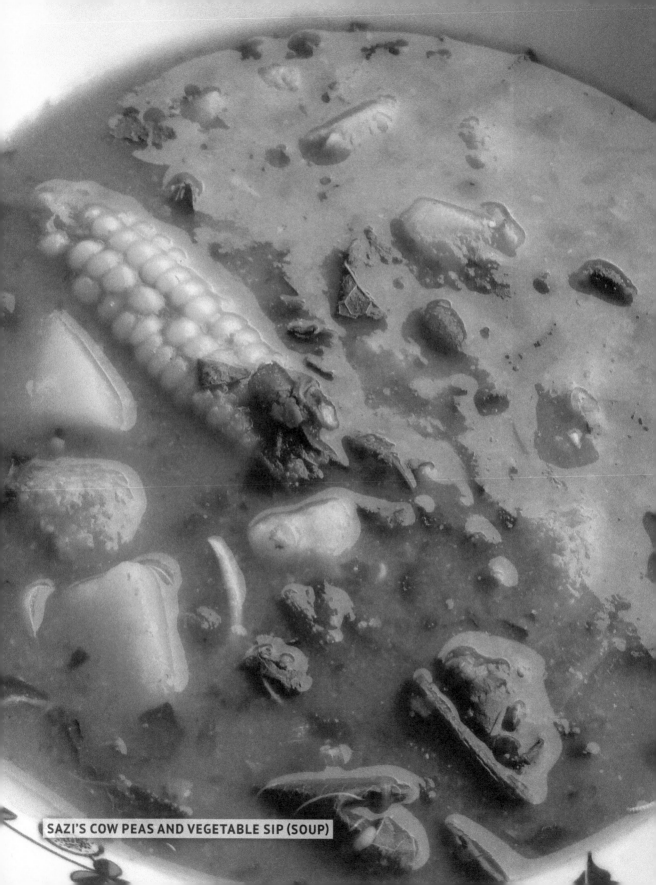

SAZI'S COW PEAS AND VEGETABLE SIP (SOUP)

Sazi's Cow Peas and Vegetable Sip (Soup)

Ingredients

200g	dried cow peas
2–3	fresh maize (corn)
200g	eddoes
150g	pumpkin fruit
50g	wholewheat flour
200g	mixed green leaves
300ml	coconut milk (optional)

escallion, thyme, pepper, pimento leaves, salt to taste

Method

Wash dried cow peas and put to boil in large saucepan. Discard the water and cover with 1 litre (4 cups) of fresh water, add salt to taste and leave to boil until tender. Wash, dice and add eddoes. Cut maize cobs into 2 or 3 and add to saucepan. Add water or coconut milk, pimento leaves, pepper, thyme and 100g pumpkin and leave to simmer.

Grate 50g pumpkin and mix with whole wheat flour, form into dumplings and add to soup. Cook for 15 minutes. Add mixed green leaves and leave on low heat for 5 minutes. Turn off heat, leave to sit for 10 minutes before serving.

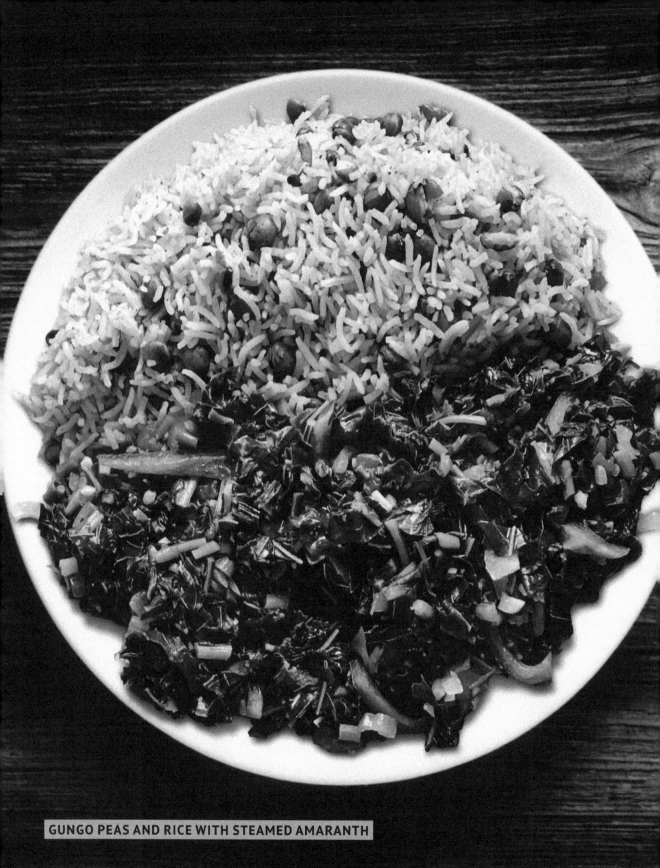

GUNGO PEAS AND RICE WITH STEAMED AMARANTH

Gungo Peas and Rice With Steamed Amaranth

Ingredients

150–200g	gungo peas
500g	rice
200ml	coconut milk

herbs, spices and salt to taste

Method

Wash the peas, cover with water and leave to boil. If dried peas are used, they need to be soaked before cooking, discard that water, add fresh water and boil until cooked but firm. If fresh gungo peas are used, these don't need to be soaked, the water doesn't need to be discarded and the cooking time will be much shorter.

Once peas are cooked, add the coconut milk, herbs and spices and salt according to preference. Wash rice, stir in cover pot and allow to cook until rice is tender, usually about 20 minutes.

Steamed Amaranth

500g	fresh amaranth
1	onion
2 medium	tomatoes
2 cloves	garlic
1	scotch bonnet pepper
20ml	oil

Strip the outer skin of the amaranth stalks, wash thoroughly and cut into small pieces. Heat the oil in a stew pot, add chopped onion, garlic and pepper. Add the finely cut tomatoes and continue frying until soft. Stir in the amaranth, add herbs, spices and salt (if desired) and leave to steam for 5–10 minutes.

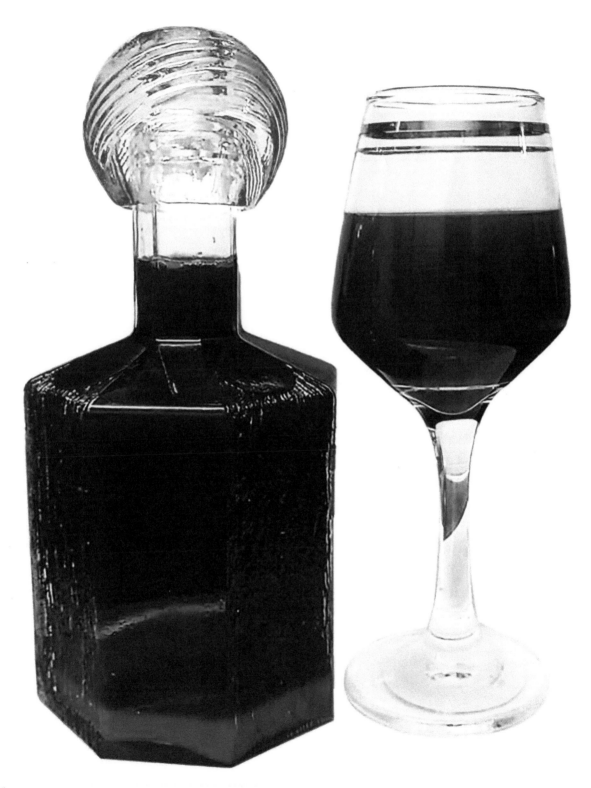

SANCHA'S SUPER SORREL DRINK (BISAP)

Sancha's Super Sorrel Drink (Bisap)

Ingredients

500g	dried sorrel calyces
200g	brown sugar
100g	ginger
5–10	dried pimento berries
5	cloves
5L	hot, just boiled water

Method

Wash sorrel and place in large saucepan or other container with tight-fitting lid. Clean and wash ginger, chop or grate and add to sorrel. Add pimento berries and cloves, cover the contents with the hot water and leave to steep for 24–36 hours. Sweeten the mixture with sugar or other sweetener (optional).

Line a fine sieve with a clean piece of muslin or similar fabric, strain the mixture into another container. Leave to sit, chill and serve.

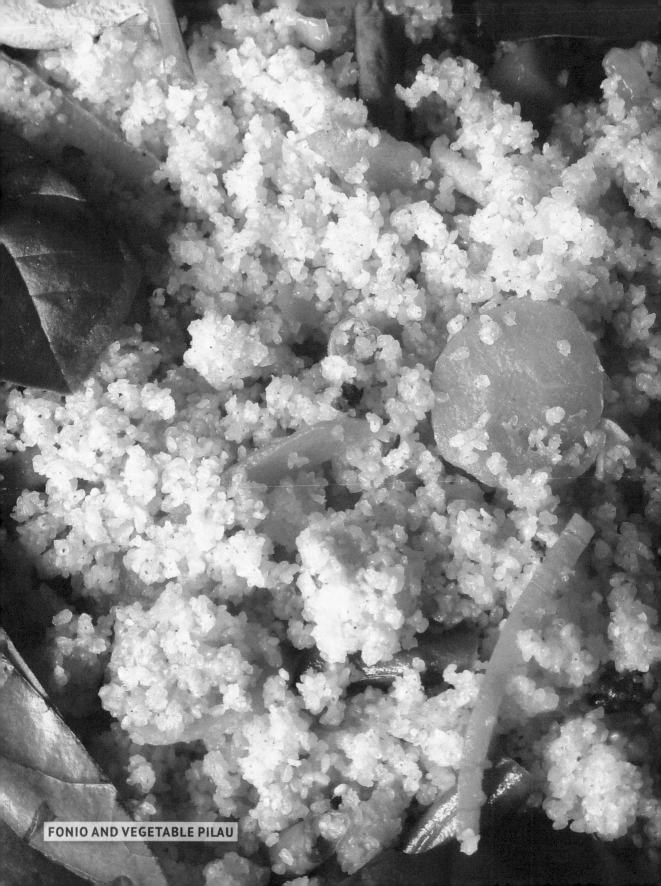

FONIO AND VEGETABLE PILAU

Fonio and Vegetable Pilau

Ingredients

200g	fonio
400ml	water or vegetable stock
1	onion
4 cloves	garlic
1	Scotch bonnet pepper
1	medium carrot
50g	green beans
1	tomato
2 tbsp	mixed spices (coriander, turmeric, cumin)
1 tbsp	mixed herbs
20ml	vegetable oil
salt to taste	

Method

Heat oil in a saucepan. Add chopped onion, garlic and pepper and fry for few minutes. Add spices and chopped tomato, cook for couple of minutes and add water or vegetable stock and salt. Cut carrot and green beans, add to mixture, add herbs and cook for a further 5 minutes.

Slowly stir in fonio grains and leave to simmer on low flame for 5–10 minutes. Turn off flame and leave to sit for 10 minutes. Serve with stew, fried ripe plantain, salad or raw greens.

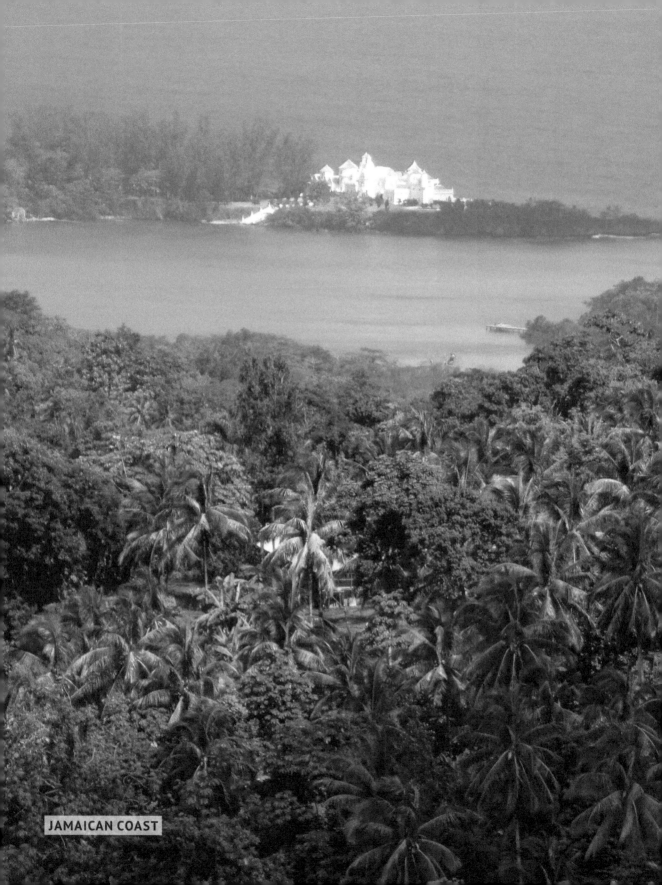

JAMAICAN COAST

References & Bibliography

Adeleke, R. O. and Abiodun, O. A. (2010) 'Nutritional Composition of Breadnut Seeds (Artocarpus camansi)', *African Journal of Agricultural Research*, 5(11), pp. 1273–76.

Agazue, O. C., Akanji, F. T., Tafida, M. A, and Kamal, M. J. (2013) 'Nutritional and some elemental composition of Shea (Vitellaria paradoxa) fruit pulp', *Archives of Applied Science Research*, 5(3), pp. 63–65.

Ballogou, V. Y., Soumanou, M. M., Toukourou F. and Hounhouigan, J. D. (2013) 'Structure and nutritional composition of fonio (Digitaria exilis) grains: a review', *International Research Journal of Biological Sciences*, 2(1), pp. 73–79.

Bamshaiye, O.M., Adegbol, J. A. and Bamishaiye, E. I. (2011) 'Bambara Groundnut: An Underutilised Nut in Africa', *Advances in Agricultural Biotechnology*, (1), pp. 60–72.

Boakye, A. A., Wireko-Manu, F. D., Oduro, I., Ellis, W. O., Gudjónsdóttir, M. and Chronakis, I. S. (2018) 'Utilizing cocoyam (Xanthosoma sagittifolium) for food and nutrition security: A review', *Food Science & Nutrition*, 13, 6(4), pp. 703–713. doi: 10.1002/fsn3.602.

British Nutrition Foundation (2021) http://www.nutrition.org.uk.

Carney, J. (2013) 'Seeds of Memory: Botanical Legacies of the African Diaspora', in Voeks, R. and Rashford, J. (eds.) *African Ethnobotany in The Americas*. New York: Springer.

CARPHA (2016) *State of Public Health in The Caribbean 2014–2016: Building Resilience to Immediate and Increasing Threats: Vector-borne Diseases and Childhood Obesity*. Port of Spain, Trinidad and Tobago: Caribbean Public Health Agency. Available at https://carpha.org/Portals/0/Documents/State-of-Public-Health-in-the-Caribbean-2014-2016.pdf.

CARPHA (2019) *State of Public Health in the Caribbean Report 2017–2018: Climate and Health: Averting and Responding to an Unfolding Health Crisis*. Port of Spain, Trinidad and Tobago: Caribbean Public Health Agency. Available at https://carpha.org/Portals/0/Documents/CARPHA_SoPH_2017_2018_Chapter_5_Responses_to_Climate_and_Health.pdf.

Cénat, J. M., McIntee and Blais-Rochette, C. (2020) 'Symptoms of posttraumatic stress disorder, depression, anxiety and other mental health problems following the 2010 earthquake in Haiti: A systematic review and meta-analysis', *Journal of Affective Disorders*, 273, 1 August 2020, pp. 55–85.

De Caluwé, E., Halanová, K. and Van Damme, P. (2010) 'Adansonia digitata L.- A review of traditional uses, phytochemistry and pharmacology', *Afrika Focus*, 23(1), pp 11–51. doi: 10.21825/af.v23i1.5037.

DebMandal, M. and Mandal, S. (2011) 'Coconut (Cocos nucifera L Aracaceae): In Health Promotion and Disease Prevention', *Asian Pacific Journal of Tropical Medicine*, 4(3), pp. 241–247. doi: 10.1016/S1995-7645(11)60078-3.

Del Rio, A. and Simpson, B. M. (2014). *Agricultural Adaptation to Climate Change in The Sahel: A Review of Fifteen Crops Cultivated in The Sahel*. USAID, African and Latin American Resilience to Climate Change (ARCC). Available at https://www.climatelinks.org/resources/agricultural-adaptation-climate-change-sahel-review-fifteen-crops-cultivated-sahel.

Dias-Martins, A. M., Pessanha, K. L. F., Pacheco, S., Rodrigues, J. A. S. and Carvalho, C. W. P. (2018). 'Potential use of pearl millet (Pennisetum glaucum). Food security, processing, health benefits, nutritional products', Food Research International, 109, pp. 175–186. doi: 10.1016/j.foodres.2018.03/023.

Duke, J. A. (1996) *Handbook of Energy Crops* (unpublished).

European Commission (2016). *Sahel: Food and Nutrition Crisis: Echo Factsheet*. July 2016. Available at http://www.ec.europa.eu/echo.

Ewing-Chow, D. (2019) 'The Environmental Impact of Caribbean tourism undermines its Economic Benefit', *Forbes Magazine*, 26 November 2019. Available at https://www.forbes.com/sites/daphneewingchow/2019/11/26/the-carbon-footprint-of-caribbean-tourism-undermines-its-economic-benefit/.

Fadl, K. E. M. (2015) 'Balanites aegyptica (L): A Multipurpose Fruit Tree in Savanna Zone of Western Sudan', *International Journal of Environment*, 4(1), pp. 197–203. doi: 10.3126/ije.v4i1.12188.

FAO and CDB (2019). *Study on the State of Agriculture in The Caribbean*. doi: 10.4060/CA4726EN.

FAO, IFAD, UNICEF, WFP and WHO (2020) *The State of Food Security and Nutrition in the World 2020: Transforming food systems for affordable healthy diets*. doi: 10.4060/ca9692en.

Fuglie, L. J. (2001) *The Moringa Tree: A local solution to malnutrition?* Dakar: Church World Service.

Gemede, H. F., Retta, N., Haki, G. D., Woldegiorgis, A. Z. and Beyene, F. (2015) 'Nutritional Quality and Health Benefits of Okra (Abelmoschus esculentus): A Review', *International Journal of Nutrition and Food Sciences*, 25(1), pp. 16-25. doi: 10.11648/j.ijnfs.20150402.22.

Gernmah, D. I., Atolagbe, M. O. and Echegwo, C. C. (2007) 'Nutritional Composition of the African Locust Bean (Parkia biglobosa) Fruit Pulp', *Nigerian Food Journal*, 25(1), pp. 190–196. doi: 10.4314/nifoj. v25i1.33669.

Global Justice Now (2015). *Growing Evidence Against the New Alliance for Food Security and Nutrition.* July 2015. Available at https://www.globaljustice.org.uk/resources/growing-evidence-against-new-alliance-food-security-and-nutrition.

Hettiaratchi, U. P. K., Ekanayake, S. and Welihinda, J. (2011) 'Natural Assessment of a Jackfruit (Artocarpus heterophyllus) Meal', *Ceylon Medical Journal*, 56(2), pp. 54–58. doi: 10.4038/cmj.v56i2.3109.

Hossain S., Ahmed R., Bhowmick S., Mamun A. A. and Hashimoto M. 'Proximate composition and fatty acid analysis of Lablab purpureus (L.) legume seed: implicates to both protein and essential fatty acid supplementation', *Springerplus*, 2016, 5(1), 1899. doi: 10.1186/s40064-016-3587-1.

Jideani, I. A. and Jideani, V. A. (2011) 'Developments on the Cereal Grains Digitaria exilis (acha) and Digitaria iburua (iburu)', *Journal of Food Science and Technology*, 48(3), pp. 251–259. doi: 10.1007/s13197-010-0208-9.

Jideani, V. A. and Diedericks, C. F. (2014) 'Nutritional, Therapeutic and Prophylactic Properties of Vigna subterranea and Moringa oleifera', *InTech*, 5 February 2014. doi: 10.5772/57338.

Karri, V. R. and Nalluri, N. (2017) 'Pigeon Pea (Cajanus cajan L) by-products as potent natural resource to produce protein rich edible food products', *International Journal of Current Agricultural Sciences*, 7(7), pp. 229–236.

Kouyaté, AM and Lamien, N. (2011) *Detarium microcarpum, sweet detar. Conservation and Sustainable Use of Genetic Resources of Priority Food Tree Species in sub-Saharan Africa.* Rome: Bioversity International. Available at https://citarea.cita-aragon.es/citarea/bitstream/10532/1687/1/2011_343EN.pdf.

Kumar, S., Tony, E., Kumar, A. P., Kumar, A., Rao, B. S. and Nadendla, R. (2013) 'A Review on Abelmoschus esculentus (Okra)', *International Research Journal of Pharmaceutical and Applied Sciences*, 3(4), pp. 129–132.

Kuru, P. (2014) 'Tamarindus indica and its health related benefits', *Asian Pacific Journal of Tropical Biomedicine*, 4(9), pp. 676–81. doi: 10.12980/APJTB.4.2014APJTB-2014-0173.

Lykke, A. M. and Padanou, E. A. (2019). 'Carbohydrates, Proteins, Fats and Other Essential Components of Food from Native Trees in West Africa', *Heliyon*, 5(5), e01744. doi: 10.1016/j.heliyon.2019.e01744.

Mazahib, A. M., Nuha, M. O., Salawa, I. S. and Babiker, E. E. (2013). 'Some Nutritional Attributes of Bambara Groundnut as Influenced by Domestic Processing', *International Food Research Journal*, 20(3), pp. 1165–71.

Mohamed, M. and Wickham, L. D. (2011) 'Breadnut (Artocarpus camansi Blanco)', in Yahia, E. M. (ed.) *Post Harvest Biology and Technology of Tropical and Subtropical Fruits. Volume 2: Açai to Citrus*. Oxford: Woodhead Publishing Limited.

Morales-Payán, J. P., Ortiz, J. R., Cicero, J. and Taveras, F. (2002). 'Digitaria exilis as a Crop in The Dominican Republic', in Janick, J. and Whipkey, A. (eds.) *Trends in New Crops and New Uses*. Alexandria, VA: ASHS Press.

Morton, J. F. (1987) 'Jackfruit', in Morton, J. (ed.) *Fruits of Warm Climates*. Miami, FL: Florida Flair Books.

Moseley, W. G. (2012). 'The Corporate Takeover of African Food Security', *Pambazuka News*, 8 November 2012. Available at https://www.pambazuka.org/food-health/corporate-take-over-african-food-security.

Muggah, R. and Luengo Cabrera, J. (2019) *The Sahel is engulfed by Violence. Climate Change, Food Insecurity and Extremists are largely to blame*. World Economic Forum, 23 January 2019. Available at https://www.weforum.org/agenda/2019/01/all-the-warning-signs-are-showing-in-the-sahel-we-must-act-now/.

National Research Council (1996) *Lost Crops of Africa: Volume I: Grains*. Washington, D.C.: National Academy Press. doi: 10.17226/2305.

National Research Council (2006) *Lost Crops of Africa: Volume II: Vegetables*. Washington, D.C.: National Academy Press. doi: 10.17226/11763

National Research Council (2008) *Lost Crops of Africa: Volume III: Fruits*. Washington, D.C.: National Academy Press. doi: 10.17226/11879.

Nourish the Planet (2011) *African Indigenous Crops*. nourishingtheplanet.org: Worldwatch Institute.

Oakland Institute (2016). *Unholy Alliance: Five Western Donors Shape a Pro-Corporate Agenda for African Agriculture*. Available at https://www.oaklandinstitute.org/five-western-donors-shape-corporate-agenda-african-agriculture.

Oibiokpa, F. I., Adoga, G. I., Saidu, A. N. and Shittu, K. O. (2014) 'Nutritional Composition of Detarium microcarpum Fruit', *African Journal of Food Science*, 8(6), pp. 342–50.

Olumakaiye, M. F. (2011) 'Evaluation of Nutrient Contents of Amaranth Leaves Prepared Using Different Coking Methods', *Food and Nutrition Sciences*, 2(4), pp. 249–252. doi: 10.4236/fns.2011.24035.

Omotesho, K. F., Sola-Ojo, F. E., Fayeye, T. R., Babatunde, R. O., Otunola, G. A. and Aliyu, T. H. (2013) 'The potential of moringa tree for poverty alleviation and rural development: Review of evidences on usage and efficacy', *International Journal of Development and Sustainability*, 2(2), pp. 799–813.

Orwa C., Mutua, A., Kindt, R., Simons, A. and Jamnadass, R. H. (2010). *Agroforestree Database: A tree reference and selection guide*. Available at https://www.worldagroforestry.org/publication/agroforestree-database-tree-reference-and-selection-guide-version-40.

Owusu-Darko, P. G., Paterson, A. and Omenyo, E. L. (2014) 'Cocoyam (corms and cormels) – An underexploited food and feed resource', *Journal of Agricultural Chemistry and Environment*, 3(1), pp. 22–29. doi: 10.4236/jacen.2014.31004.

Popova, A. and Mihaylova, D. (2019) 'Antinutrients in Plant-based Foods: A Review', The Open Biotechnology Journal, 15, pp. 68–76. doi: 10.2174/1874070701913010068.

Quarless, D. (2020) *Sustainable Responses for a Post-Covid19 Economic Recovery*. Virtual Meeting for Parliamentarians of the Americas and The Caribbean, 11 June 2020. Available at https://parlamericas.org/uploads/documents/Agenda_Economic_Recovery_ENG.pdf.

Rashmi D. R., Raghu N., Gopenath T. S., Pradeep P., Pugazhandhi B., Murugesan K., Ashok G., Ranjith M. S., Chandrashekrappa G. K. and Kanthesh, M. B. (2018) 'Taro (Colocasia esculenta): An Overview', *Journal of Medicinal Plants Studies*. 6(4), pp. 156–161.

Sagna, M. B., Diallo, A., Sarr, P. S., Ndiaye, O., Goffner, D. and Guisse, A. (2014) 'Biochemical Composition and Nutritional Value of Balanites aegyptica (L) Del Fruit Pulp from Northern Ferlo Senegal', *African Journal of Biotechnology*, 13(2), pp. 336–42.

Santos, A. C. P., Alves, A. M., Naves, M. M. V. and Silva, M. (2020) 'Nutritional profile, bioactive compounds and antioxidant capacity of jatobá-da-mata (Hymenaea courbaril) by product', *Revista Chilena de Nutricion*, 47(3), pp. 366–371. doi: 10.4067/S0717-751820000300366.

Scaling Up Nutrition. (2018). *Making Nutrition a Political and Financial Priority in The Sahel and West Africa*. Conclusions from Conference, 13 December 2018. Available at https://scalingupnutrition.org/news/making-nutrition-a-political-and-financial-priority-in-the-sahel-and-west-africa/.

Sharma, S. and Ramana Rao, T. V. (2013) 'Nutritional quality characteristics of pumpkin fruit as revealed by its biochemical analysis', *International Food Research Journal*, 20(5), pp. 2309–16.

Sharma, S., Agarwal, N. and Verma, P. (2011) 'Pigeon Pea (Cajanus cajan L): A Hidden Treasure of Nutrition Regime', *Journal of Functional and Environmental Botany*, 1(2), pp. 91–101. doi: 10.5958/j.2231-1742.1.2.010.

Shukla, A., Lalit, A., Sharma, V., Vats, S. and Alam, A. (2015) 'Pearl and Finger Millets: The Hope of Food Security', *Applied Research Journal*, 1(2), pp. 59–66.

Sidibe, M. and Williams, J. T. (2002) *Baobab, Adansonia digitata*. Southampton: University of Southampton, International Centre for Underutilised Crops.

Singh, P., Khan, M. and Hailemariam, H. (2017) 'Nutritional and Health Importance of Hibiscus sabdariffa: A Review and Indication for Research Needs', *Journal of Nutritional Health & Food Engineering*, 6(5), pp. 125–128.

Sonkin, F. (2018). *Two Blows in a Row: The New Alliance for Food Security Loses Ground*. Oakland Institute. Available at https://www.oaklandinstitute.org/blog/two-blows-row-new-alliance-food-security-loses-ground.

Soriano-García, M. and Aguirre-Díaz, I. S. (2019) 'Nutritional Functional Value and Therapeutic Utilization of Amaranth', *InTech*, 29 August 2019. doi: 10.5772/intechopen.86897.

Suresh, S. and Sisodia, S. S. (2018) 'Phytochemical and Pharmacological Aspects of Cucurbita moschata and Moringa oleifera', *UK Journal of Pharmaceutical and Biosciences*, 6(6), pp. 45–53.

Swanevelder, C. J. (1998) *Bambara – Food for Africa (Vigna subterranea–bambara groundnut)*. National Department of Agriculture, ARC-LNR. Available at https://www.nda.agric.za/docs/brochures/bambara.pdf.

Temesgen, M. and Ratta, N. (2017). 'Nutritional potential, Health and Food Security Benefits of Taro Colocasia esculenta (L.): A Review', *The Open Food Science Journal*, June 2015. Available at http://www.researchgate.net/publication/318562639.

Useful Tropical Plants Database (2019) *Hymenaea Courbaril*. Available at http://tropical.theferns.info/viewtropical.php?id=Hymenaea+courbaril.

Washington State University (2021) *myNutrition*. Available at http://www.mynutrition.wsu.edu/.

Index

Lightning Source UK Ltd.
Milton Keynes UK
UKHW050901101021
391922UK00003B/10